Student Workbook

to Accompany

Health Science Career Exploration

Student Workbook

to Accompany

Health Science Career Exploration

Louise Simmers, MEd, RN

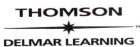

THOMSON

DELMAR LEARNING

Australia   Canada   Mexico   Singapore   Spain   United Kingdom   United States

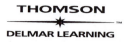

THOMSON
————★———— ™
DELMAR LEARNING

Student Workbook to Accompany Health Science Career Exploration
By Louise Simmers

Vice President, Health Care Business Unit:
William Brottmiller

Editorial Director:
Cathy L. Esperti

Acquisitions Editor:
Marah Bellegarde

Developmental Editor:
Debra Flis

Editorial Assistant:
Erin Adams

Marketing Director:
Jennifer McAvey

Marketing Channel Manager:
Tamara Caruso

Project Editor:
Natalie Wager

Senior Art/Design Coordinator:
Connie Lundberg-Watkins

Production Editor:
Anne Sherman

COPYRIGHT © 2004 by Delmar Learning, a division of Thomson Learning, Inc. Thomson Learning™ is a trademark used herein under license.

Printed in the United States of America
  6 7 8 9 XXX 09 08 07

For more information, contact Delmar Learning, 5 Maxwell Drive, Clifton Park, NY 12065
Or find us on the World Wide Web at http://www.delmarlearning.com

Library of Congress Cataloging-in-Publication Number:

2003024038

ISBN 13: 978-1-4018-5812-4
ISBN 10: 1-4018-5812-0

CONTENTS

To the Student vii

Matrix of Skills Used in Health Occupations and Correlation to National Health Care Standards ix

| CHAPTER 1 | HISTORY AND TRENDS OF HEALTH CARE . . . . | 1 |
| | Internet Searches . . . . | 4 |

| CHAPTER 2 | HEALTH CARE SYSTEMS . . . . | 5 |
| | Internet Searches . . . . | 7 |

| CHAPTER 3 | PERSONAL QUALITIES OF A HEALTH CARE WORKER . . . . | 9 |
| | Internet Searches . . . . | 13 |

CHAPTER 4	CAREERS IN HEALTH CARE	15
4:1	Careers in Health Care	15
4:2	Demonstrating Brushing and Flossing Techniques	19
	A Demonstrating Brushing Techniques . . .	21
	B Demonstrating Flossing Techniques	23
4:3	Operating the Microscope	26
4:4	Administering Oxygen	34
4:5	Completing a Statistical Data Sheet	41
4:6	Admitting a Patient	48
4:7	Measuring/Recording Height and Weight . .	56
4:8	Part 1: Mental Health Myths Test	62
	Part 2: How Do Others See You?	65
4:9	Writing an Obituary	69
4:10	Transferring a Patient to a Wheelchair	71
4:11	Feeding a Patient	77
4:12	Ambulating a Patient with Crutches	83
4:13	Applying a Moist Compress	91
4:14	Screening for Vision Problems	97
	Internet Searches	102

| CHAPTER 5 | LEGAL AND ETHICAL RESPONSIBILITIES . . . . | 103 |
| | Internet Searches . . . . | 107 |

| CHAPTER 6 | CULTURAL DIVERSITY . . . . | 109 |
| | Internet Searches . . . . | 114 |

CHAPTER 7	MEDICAL TERMINOLOGY	115
7:1	Using Medical Abbreviations	115
7:2	Interpreting Word Parts	118
	Internet Searches	122

| CHAPTER 8 | MEDICAL MATH . . . . | 123 |
| | Internet Searches . . . . | 125 |

| CHAPTER 9 | COMPUTERS IN HEALTH CARE . . . . | 127 |
| | Internet Searches . . . . | 128 |

CHAPTER 10	PROMOTION OF SAFETY	129
10:1	Using Body Mechanics	129
10:2	Preventing Accidents and Injuries	132
10:3	Observing Fire Safety	137
	Safety Examination	141
	Internet Searches	144

CHAPTER 11	INFECTION CONTROL	145
11:1	Understanding the Principles of Infection Control	145
11:2	Washing Hands	148
11:3	Observing Standard Precautions	151
11:4	Maintaining Transmission-Based Isolation Precautions	157
	Donning and Removing Transmission-Based Isolation Garments	159
11:5	Bioterrorism	163
	Internet Searches	164

CHAPTER 12	VITAL SIGNS	165
12:1	Measuring and Recording Vital Signs	165
12:2	Measuring and Recording Temperature	167
	A Measuring and Recording Oral Temperature with a Clinical Thermometer	170
	B Measuring Oral Temperature with an Electronic Thermometer	173
	C Measuring and Recording Tympanic (Aural) Temperature	175
12:3	Measuring and Recording Pulse	178
12:4	Measuring and Recording Respirations	181
12:5	Measuring and Recording Apical Pulse	184
12:6	Measuring and Recording Blood Pressure . .	187
	Reading a Mercury Sphygmomanometer . . .	189
	Reading an Aneroid Sphygmomanometer . .	190
	Internet Searches	194

CHAPTER 13	FIRST AID	195
13:1	Providing First Aid	195
13:2	Performing Cardiopulmonary Resuscitation (CPR)	197
	A One-Person Rescue	199
	B Infants	202
	C Children	205
	D Obstructed Airway on Conscious Adult Victim	208
	E Obstructed Airway on Unconscious Victim	210
13:3	Providing First Aid for Bleeding and Wounds	214
13:4	Providing First Aid for Shock	220
13:5	Providing First Aid for Poisoning	225
13:6	Providing First Aid for Burns	230
13:7	Providing First Aid for Heat Exposure	235
13:8	Providing First Aid for Cold Exposure	240

13:9   Providing First Aid for Bone and
        Joint Injuries 243
13:10   Providing First Aid for Specific Injuries . . . 250
13:11   Providing First Aid for Sudden Illness 258
13:12   Applying Dressings and Bandages 264
        Internet Searches 270

**CHAPTER 14 PREPARING FOR THE WORLD
                    OF WORK** 271
14:1   Developing Job-Keeping Skills 271
14:2   Writing a Letter of Application and
        Preparing a Resumé 272

        Inventory Sheet for Resumés 274
14:3   Completing Job Application Forms 278
        Wallet Card 279
        Sample Form 280
14:4   Participating in a Job Interview 284
14:5   Determining Net Income 287
14:6   Calculating a Budget 291
        Internet Searches 294

INDEX 295

To the Student

Three types of worksheets are provided in this workbook: assignment sheets, procedure sheets, and evaluation sheets. These sheets are designed to correlate with specific information discussed in the textbook, *Health Science Career Exploration*.

The assignment sheets are designed to allow you to review the main facts and information about a procedure. After you read the information about a specific procedure, try to answer the questions on the corresponding assignment sheet. Refer to the information in the text to obtain the correct answers to the questions or statements. Then check the information to be sure your answers are correct. Let your instructor grade the completed assignment sheet. Note any points that are not correct. Be sure you understand these points before you perform the procedure. This practice will provide you with the basic knowledge or facts necessary before a procedure is done.

The procedure sheets provide step-by-step directions for performing specific tasks. The word *Note* in the procedure stresses when important information is provided about a specific step in the procedure. The word *Caution* means a safety point is involved. Legal responsibilities are stressed by the presence of the legal icon. Communication points are stressed by the communication icon. At the end of each procedure, a student alert will tell you to use an evaluation sheet to practice the procedure. By reading all of the steps in the procedure sheet and practicing the procedure with the evaluation sheet, you will learn to do the specific skill correctly and safely. (See Icon Key below.)

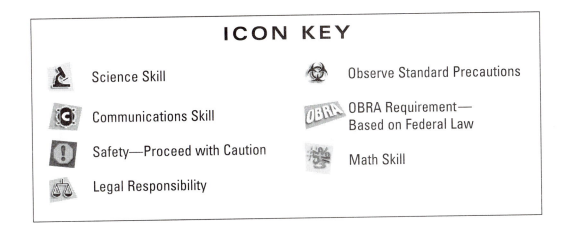

The evaluation sheets are designed to set criteria or standards that should be observed while a specific procedure is being performed. They follow the steps of the procedure as listed in the procedure sections. As you practice each procedure, use the specific evaluation sheet to judge your performance. When you feel you have mastered a particular procedure, sign the evaluation sheet and give it to your instructor. The instructor will use this sheet to grade your performance.

The format of the evaluation sheet is designed to provide for both practice and the final evaluation of the procedure. The appearance of the evaluation sheet and the meaning of each of the abbreviations and parts are as follows:

EVALUATION SHEET

Name _____ Date _____

Evaluated by _____

DIRECTIONS:

Name of Procedure	Points Possible	Yes	No	Points Earned	Comments

Name: Sign your name in this area.

Date: The date you are given your final evaluation can be placed in this area.

Evaluated by: The person who is evaluating you (usually the instructor) on your final check of this procedure will sign his or her name in this area.

Directions: Basic directions for using the sheet are provided in this area.

Name of Procedure: The specific name of the procedure will be noted in this area.

Points Possible: A number will appear in this column beside each step of the procedure. The number represents the points you will receive if you do this step of the procedure correctly.

Yes/No: These columns will be used by the person (usually the instructor) doing your final check or evaluation on the procedure. If you perform a step of the procedure correctly, the evaluator will place a check in the "Yes" column. If you do not perform a step of the procedure, or perform a step incorrectly, the evaluator will place a check in the "No" column.

Points Earned: In this column the evaluator will give you the correct number of points (as stated in the "Points Possible" column) for each step of the procedure on which you received a check in the "Yes" column. You will not receive the points for a particular step if you received a check in the "No" column. The number of points earned can then be totaled. A grade can be assigned by a scale determined by your instructor.

Comments: This column is for comments regarding your performance of the procedure. Any check in the "No" column should be explained by a brief explanation opposite the step in which the error occurred. In addition, positive comments on your performance of the procedure should be noted in this area.

As you can see, the evaluation sheet provides you with an opportunity to actually practice your performance test on a particular procedure before you have to take the final performance evaluation. By utilizing this sheet, you will achieve higher standards of performance and learn to master all steps of each procedure.

The sheets in this book follow the same order of procedures and skills found in the textbook. Each information section in the textbook refers you to a specific assignment sheet in the workbook. Each procedure section in the workbook has a specific evaluation sheet. By using the information in the textbook and following the directions on each of the sheets in this workbook, you can master the procedures and skills and become a competent health care worker.

Matrix of Skills Used in Health Occupations and Correlation to National Health Care Skill Standards

Matrix of Skills Used In Health Occupations

SKILLS	CLINICAL LABORATORY SERVICES	DENTISTRY	DIETETICS AND NUTRITION	EDUCATION	HEALTH INFORMATION AND COMMUNICATION	HEALTH SERVICES ADMINISTRATION	MEDICINE	MENTAL, PHYSICAL SOCIAL SPECIALTIES	NURSING	PHARMACY	PODIATRY	SCIENCE AND ENGINEERING	TECHNICAL INSTRUMENTATION	VETERINARY MEDICINE	VISION CARE
Chapter 1: History and Trends of Health Care															
History of health care	X	X	X	X	X	X	X	X	X	X	X	X	X	X	X
Trends in health care	X	X	X	X	X	X	X	X	X	X	X	X	X	X	X
Chapter 2: Health Care Systems															
Private health care facilities	X	X	X	X	X	X	X	X	X	X	X	X	X	X	X
Government agencies	X	X	X	X	X	X	X	X	X	X	X	X	X	X	X
Voluntary or nonprofit agencies	X	X	X	X	X	X	X	X	X	X	X	X	X	X	X
Health insurance plans	X	X	X	X	X	X	X	X	X	X	X	X	X	X	X
Organizational structure	X	X	X	X	X	X	X	X	X	X	X	X	X	X	X
Chapter 3: Personal Qualities of a Health Care Worker															
Personal appearance	X	X	X	X	X	X	X	X	X	X	X	X	X	X	X
Personal characteristics	X	X	X	X	X	X	X	X	X	X	X	X	X	X	X
Effective communications	X	X	X	X	X	X	X	X	X	X	X	X	X	X	X
Teamwork	X	X	X	X	X	X	X	X	X	X	X	X	X	X	X
Professional leadership	X	X	X	X	X	X	X	X	X	X	X	X	X	X	X
Stress	X	X	X	X	X	X	X	X	X	X	X	X	X	X	X
Time management	X	X	X	X	X	X	X	X	X	X	X	X	X	X	X
Chapter 4: Careers in Health Care															
Introduction to health careers	X	X	X	X	X	X	X	X	X	X	X	X	X	X	X
Dental careers		X		X											
Diagnostic services	X	X	X	X	X	X	X	X	X	X	X	X	X	X	X
Emergency medical services	X	X	X	X	X	X	X	X	X	X	X	X	X	X	X
Health information and communication services	X	X	X	X	X	X	X	X	X	X	X	X	X	X	X
Hospital/health care facility services	X		X	X	X	X	X	X	X	X	X				
Medical careers				X		X	X		X		X				X
Mental and social services				X	X	X	X	X	X						
Mortuary careers				X	X	X	X	X	X						
Nursing careers				X	X	X	X		X			X			
Nutrition and dietary services		X	X	X	X	X	X	X	X						
Therapeutic services	X	X	X	X	X	X	X	X	X	X	X	X	X	X	X
Veterinary careers				X	X									X	
Vision services				X	X	X	X	X	X	X			X		X
Chapter 5: Legal and Ethical Responsibilities															
Legal responsibilities	X	X	X	X	X	X	X	X	X	X	X	X	X	X	X
Eth ́cs	X	X	X	X	X	X	X	X	X	X	X	X	X	X	X
Patient's rights	X	X	X	X	X	X	X	X	X	X	X	X	X	X	X
Advance directives for health care	X	X	X	X	X	X	X	X	X	X	X	X	X	X	X
Professional standards	X	X	X	X	X	X	X	X	X	X	X	X	X	X	X

Matrix of Skills Used In Health Occupations

SKILLS	CLINICAL LABORATORY SERVICES	DENTISTRY	DIETETICS AND NUTRITION	EDUCATION	HEALTH INFORMATION AND COMMUNICATION	HEALTH SERVICES ADMINISTRATION	MEDICINE	MENTAL, PHYSICAL SOCIAL SPECIALTIES	NURSING	PHARMACY	PODIATRY	SCIENCE AND ENGINEERING	TECHNICAL INSTRUMENTATION	VETERINARY MEDICINE	VISION CARE
Chapter 6: Cultural Diversity															
Culture, ethnicity, and race	X	X	X	X	X	X	X	X	X	X	X	X	X	X	X
Bias, prejudice, and stereotyping	X	X	X	X	X	X	X	X	X	X	X	X	X	X	X
Understanding cultural diversity	X	X	X	X	X	X	X	X	X	X	X	X	X	X	X
Respecting cultural diversity	X	X	X	X	X	X	X	X	X	X	X	X	X	X	X
Chapter 7: Medical Terminology															
Using medical abbreviations	X	X	X	X	X	X	X	X	X	X	X	X	X	X	X
Interpreting word parts	X	X	X	X	X	X	X	X	X	X	X	X	X	X	X
Chapter 8: Medical math															
Basic calculations	X	X	X	X	X	X	X	X	X	X	X	X	X	X	X
Estimating	X	X	X	X	X	X	X	X	X	X	X	X	X	X	X
Roman numerals	X	X	X	X	X	X	X	X	X	X	X	X	X	X	X
Angles	X	X	X	X	X	X	X	X	X	X	X	X	X	X	X
Systems of measurement	X	X	X	X	X	X	X	X	X	X	X	X	X	X	X
Temperature conversion	X	X	X	X	X	X	X	X	X	X	X	X	X	X	X
Military time	X	X	X	X	X	X	X	X	X	X	X	X	X	X	X
Chapter 9: Computers in Health Care															
Introduction to computers	X	X	X	X	X	X	X	X	X	X	X	X	X	X	X
What is a computer system?	X	X	X	X	X	X	X	X	X	X	X	X	X	X	X
Computer applications	X	X	X	X	X	X	X	X	X	X	X	X	X	X	X
Using the Internet	X	X	X	X	X	X	X	X	X	X	X	X	X	X	X
Communication	X	X	X	X	X	X	X	X	X	X	X	X	X	X	X
Chapter 10: Promotion of Safety															
Using body mechanics	X	X	X	X	X	X	X	X	X	X	X	X	X	X	X
Preventing accidents and injuries	X	X	X	X	X	X	X	X	X	X	X	X	X	X	X
Observing fire safety	X	X	X	X	X	X	X	X	X	X	X	X	X	X	X
CHAPTER 11: Infection Control															
Understanding the principles of infection control	X	X	X	X	X	X	X	X	X	X	X	X	X	X	X
Washing hands	X	X	X	X	X	X	X	X	X	X	X	X	X	X	X
Observing standard precautions	X	X	X	X	X	X	X	X	X	X	X	X	X	X	X
Maintaining transmission-based isolation precautions	X	X	X	X		X	X	X	X	X	X	X	X	X	X
Bioterrorism	X	X	X	X	X	X	X	X	X	X	X	X	X	X	X

Matrix of Skills Used In Health Occupations

SKILLS	CLINICAL LABORATORY SERVICES	DENTISTRY	DIETETICS AND NUTRITION	EDUCATION	HEALTH INFORMATION AND COMMUNICATION	HEALTH SERVICES ADMINISTRATION	MEDICINE	MENTAL, PHYSICAL SOCIAL SPECIALTIES	NURSING	PHARMACY	PODIATRY	SCIENCE AND ENGINEERING	TECHNICAL INSTRUMENTATION	VETERINARY MEDICINE	VISION CARE
Chapter 12: Vital Signs															
Measuring and recording vital signs	X	X		X			X	X	X	X	X	X	X	X	X
Measuring and recording temperature	X	X		X			X	X	X	X	X	X	X	X	X
Measuring and recording pulse	X	X		X			X	X	X	X	X	X	X	X	X
Measuring and recording respirations	X	X		X			X	X	X	X	X	X	X	X	X
Measuring and recording apical pulse	X	X		X			X	X	X	X	X	X	X	X	X
Measuring and recording blood pressure	X	X		X			X	X	X	X	X	X	X	X	X
Chapter 13: First Aid															
Providing first aid	X	X	X	X	X	X	X	X	X	X	X	X	X	X	X
Performing cardiopulmonary resuscitation	X	X	X	X	X	X	X	X	X	X	X	X	X	X	X
Providing first aid for bleeding and wounds	X	X	X	X	X	X	X	X	X	X	X	X	X	X	X
Providing first aid for shock	X	X	X	X	X	X	X	X	X	X	X	X	X	X	X
Providing first aid for poisoning	X	X	X	X	X	X	X	X	X	X	X	X	X	X	X
Providing first aid for burns	X	X	X	X	X	X	X	X	X	X	X	X	X	X	X
Providing first aid for heat exposure	X	X	X	X	X	X	X	X	X	X	X	X	X	X	X
Providing first aid for cold exposure	X	X	X	X	X	X	X	X	X	X	X	X	X	X	X
Providing first aid for bone and joint injuries	X	X	X	X	X	X	X	X	X	X	X	X	X	X	X
Providing first aid for specific injuries	X	X	X	X	X	X	X	X	X	X	X	X	X	X	X
Providing first aid for sudden illness	X	X	X	X	X	X	X	X	X	X	X	X	X	X	X
Applying dressings and bandages	X	X	X	X	X	X	X	X	X	X	X	X	X	X	X
Chapter 14: Preparing for the World of Work															
Developing job-keeping skills	X	X	X	X	X	X	X	X	X	X	X	X	X	X	X
Writing a letter of application and preparing a resumé	X	X	X	X	X	X	X	X	X	X	X	X	X	X	X
Completing job application forms	X	X	X	X	X	X	X	X	X	X	X	X	X	X	X
Participating in a job interview	X	X	X	X	X	X	X	X	X	X	X	X	X	X	X
Determining net income	X	X	X	X	X	X	X	X	X	X	X	X	X	X	X
Calculating a budget	X	X	X	X	X	X	X	X	X	X	X	X	X	X	X

Correlation to National Health Care Standards

CHAPTER	Health Care Core Standard								Therapeutic/ Diagnostic Core					Therapeutic Cluster			
	Academic Foundation	Communication	Systems	Employability Skills	Legal Responsibilities	Ethics	Safety Practices	Teamwork	Health Maintenance Practices	Client Interaction	Intrateam Communication	Monitoring Client Status	Client Movement	Data Collection	Treatment Planning	Implementing Procedures	Client Status Evaluation
Chapter 1	X			X													
Chapter 2	X	X	X	X	X		X	X	X		X						
Chapter 3	X	X	X	X	X	X	X	X	X	X	X						
Chapter 4	X		X	X	X			X			X			X			
Chapter 5		X	X	X	X	X				X	X	X		X	X	X	
Chapter 6	X	X		X	X	X		X	X	X	X	X	X	X	X	X	X
Chapter 7	X	X															
Chapter 8	X			X										X	X	X	X
Chapter 9	X	X		X	X						X			X			X
Chapter 10				X			X				X	X	X	X	X	X	X
Chapter 11	X			X	X	X			X		X			X		X	X
Chapter 12	X			X			X		X	X	X	X		X		X	X
Chapter 13				X	X	X				X	X	X	X	X	X	X	X
Chapter 14	X	X		X	X	X		X		X							

xiii

Correlation to National Health Care Standards

CHAPTER	Diagnostic Cluster					Information Services Cluster					Environmental Services Cluster			
	Planning	Preparation	Procedure	Evaluation	Reporting	Analysis	Abstracting and Coding	Information Systems	Documentation	Operations	Environmental Operations	Aseptic Procedures	Resource Management	Aesthetics
Chapter 1						X							X	
Chapter 2						X							X	
Chapter 3												X		
Chapter 4	X									X	X			
Chapter 5	X				X	X		X	X		X	X		
Chapter 6	X	X	X	X	X	X		X	X				X	
Chapter 7					X		X		X					
Chapter 8			X			X	X	X	X	X			X	
Chapter 9					X	X		X	X	X			X	
Chapter 10	X	X	X	X	X						X			X
Chapter 11		X	X								X	X	X	
Chapter 12	X	X	X	X	X		X		X		X			
Chapter 13	X	X	X	X	X									
Chapter 14													X	

ASSIGNMENT SHEET

Grade _____ Name _____

INTRODUCTION: Knowledge of the history of health care and an awareness of trends in health care are important for any health care worker. This assignment will help you become familiar with the history of medicine and will introduce you to the current trends in the health care field.

INSTRUCTIONS: Read the information on History and Trends of Health Care. Then follow the instructions in each section to complete this assignment.

A. Completion or Short Answer: In the space provided, print the word(s) that best completes the statement or answers the question.

   1. Describe what is meant by the following trends in health care. Include a brief explanation of why it is important to be aware of these trends.

      a. cost containment:

      b. energy conservation:

      c. home health care:

      d. geriatric care:

      e. telemedicine:

      f. wellness:

g. alternative and complementary methods of health care:

2. What is holistic health care?

3. The Omnibus Budget Reconciliation Act (OBRA) of 1987 established standards for geriatric assistants in long-term care facilities. List three (3) requirements that all geriatric assistants must meet as a result of OBRA.

4. Review Table 1-8 on alternative and complementary therapies. Name one (1) therapy you would like to try. Why do you think it would work?

5. Do you think a national health care plan should be established to provide coverage for all individuals? Why or why not?

B. Matching: Place the letter of the answer from Column B in the space provided next to the correct description in Column A.

Part I. Ancient Times

Column A	Column B
____ 1. Began public health and sanitation systems	A. Chinese
____ 2. The father of medicine	B. Egyptians
____ 3. Earliest people known to maintain accurate health records	C. Claudis Galen
____ 4. Used acupuncture to relieve pain and congestion	D. Hippocrates
____ 5. Physician who believed the body is regulated by four fluids or humors	E. Romans

Part II. Dark Ages to Renaissance

Column A	Column B
____ 1. Artist who used dissection to draw the human body	A. Leonardo da Vinci
____ 2. Emphasis was placed on saving the soul, and study of medicine was prohibited	B. Dark Ages
____ 3. An Arab physician who began the use of animal gut for suture material	C. Renaissance
____ 4. Rebirth of the science of medicine	D. Rhazes
____ 5. Published first anatomy book	E. Andreas Vesalius

Part III. 16th to 18th Century

Column A	Column B
____ 1. Developed a vaccine for smallpox in 1796	A. Gabriel Fahrenheit
____ 2. Described the circulation of blood to and from the heart	B. William Harvey
____ 3. Created the first mercury thermometer	C. Edward Jenner
____ 4. Called father of modern surgery	D. Ambrose Pare
____ 5. Invented the microscope	E. Anton Van Leeuwenhoek

Part IV. 19th Century

Column A	Column B
____ 1. Established the patterns of heredity	A. Joseph Lister
____ 2. Discovered X-rays in 1895	B. Gregory Mendel
____ 3. Began pasteurizing milk to kill bacteria	C. Florence Nightingale
____ 4. Founder of modern nursing	D. Louis Pasteur
____ 5. Began using disinfectants and antiseptics during surgery	E. William Roentgen

Part V. 20th Century

Column A

_____ 1. Isolated radium in 1910

_____ 2. Discovered penicillin in 1928

_____ 3. Developed the polio vaccine in 1952

_____ 4. Performed first successful heart transplant

_____ 5. Described how DNA carries genetic material

Column B

A. Christian Barnard

B. Francis Crick and James Watson

C. Marie Curie

D. Sir Alexander Fleming

E. Jonas Salk

CHAPTER 1 INTERNET SEARCHES

Use the suggested search engines in Chapter 9:4 of the textbook to search the Internet for additional information on the following topics:

1. _History of health care:_ Research individual names or discoveries such as the polio vaccine to gain more insight into how major developments in health care occurred.

2. _Trends in health care:_ Research topics such as home health care, Omnibus Budget Reconciliation Act of 1987, telemedicine, holistic health care, cost containment, geriatric care, and wellness to obtain additional information on the present effect on health care.

3. _Alternative/complementary methods of health care:_ Search the Internet for additional information on specific therapies such as acupuncture. Refer to Table 1-8 for a list of many different therapies.

CHAPTER 2 HEALTH CARE SYSTEMS

ASSIGNMENT SHEET

Grade _____ Name _____

INTRODUCTION: An awareness of the many different kinds of health care systems is important for any health care worker. This assignment will help you review the main facts on health care systems.

INSTRUCTIONS: Read the information on Health Care Systems. Then follow the instructions by each section to complete this assignment.

A. Completion or Short Answer: In the space provided, print the word(s) that best completes the statement or answers the question.

1. Unscramble the following words to identify some health care facilities.

    a. RAALOTBYRO

    b. OLGN ETMR AREC

    c. MNCEGEREY AECR

    d. LNCCII

    e. EAIINRIABHTLTO

    f. POTSAHIL

2. Place the name of the type of health care facility by the brief description of the facility.

    a. _____ provide assistance and care for mainly elderly patients

    b. _____ provide special care for victims of accidents or sudden illness

    c. _____ deal with mental disorders and disease

    d. _____ perform special diagnostic tests

    e. _____ provide care in a patient's home

    f. _____ provide physical, occupational, and other therapies

3. How is a general hospital different from a specialty hospital?

4. List three (3) services offered by medical offices.

5. Identify at least three (3) types of clinics.

6. List three (3) examples of services that can be provided by home health care agencies.

7. What is the purpose or main goal for the care provided by rehabilitation facilities?

8. Identify three (3) services offered by school health services.

9. An international agency sponsored by the United Nations is the _____.
   A national agency that deals with health problems in the United States is the _____.
   Another national organization that is involved in research on disease is the _____.
   A federal agency that establishes and enforces standards that protect workers from job-related injuries and illnesses is the _____.
   The federal agency that researches the quality of health care delivery and identifies the standards of treatment that should be provided is the _____.

10. Nonprofit or voluntary agencies provide many services.
    a. How do these agencies receive their funding?

    b. List two (2) services provided by these facilities.

11. Define the following terms related to insurance plans.
    a. deductible:
    b. 75/25% co-insurance:
    c. co-payment:
    d. HMOs:
    e. PPOs:

12. a. What is one advantage of HMOs?

   b. What is one disadvantage of HMOs?

13. Identify the individuals who are usually covered under the following plans.

   Medicare:

   Medicaid:

   State Children's Health Insurance Program:

   Workers' Compensation:

14. What is the purpose of an organizational structure in a health care facility?

CHAPTER 2 INTERNET SEARCHES

Use the suggested search engines in Chapter 9:4 of the textbook to search the Internet for additional information on the following topics:

1. *Private health care facilities:* Search for information on each of the specific types of facilities; for example, hospitals, hospice care, or emergency care services.

2. *Government agencies:* Search for detailed information about the activities of the World Health Organization, U.S. Department of Health and Human Services, National Institutes of Health, Centers for Disease Control and Prevention, Food and Drug Administration, and Occupational Safety and Health Administration.

3. *Voluntary or nonprofit agencies:* Search for information on the purposes and activities of organizations such as the American Cancer Society, American Heart Association, American Respiratory Disease Association, American Diabetes Association, National Association of Mental Health, National Foundation of the March of Dimes, and the American Red Cross.

4. *Health insurance:* Search the Internet to find specific names of companies that are health maintenance organizations or preferred provider organizations. Check to see how their coverage for individuals is the same or how it is different.

5. *Government health care insurance:* Search the Internet to learn about benefits provided under Medicare, Medicaid, and the State Children's Health Insurance Program.

CHAPTER 3 PERSONAL QUALITIES OF A HEALTH CARE WORKER

ASSIGNMENT SHEET

Grade _____ Name _____

INTRODUCTION: Certain personal characteristics, attitudes, and rules of appearance apply to all health care workers even though they may be employed in many different careers. This assignment will help you review these basic requirements.

INSTRUCTIONS: Read the information on Personal Qualities of a Health Care Worker. Then follow the instructions by each section and complete this assignment.

A. Crossword: Use the Key Terms for personal characteristics of a health care worker to complete the crossword puzzle.

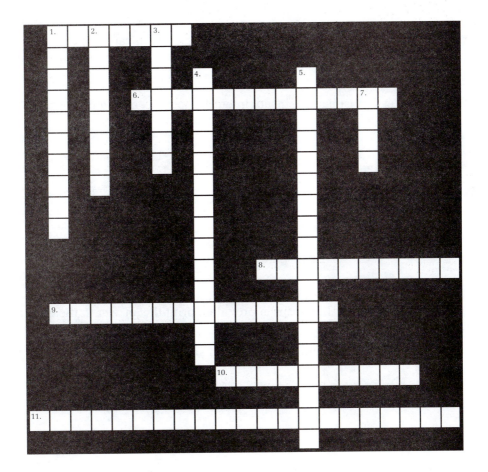

ACROSS

1. Identify with and understand another's feelings
6. Accept responsibility because others rely on you
8. Use good judgment in what you say and do
9. Willing to be held accountable for your actions
10. Qualified and capable of performing a task
11. Accept opinions of others and learn from them

DOWN

1. Display a positive attitude and enjoy work
2. Tolerant and understanding
3. Show truthfulness and integrity
4. Ability to begin or follow through with a task
5. Adapt to changes and learn new things
7. Say or do the kindest or most fitting thing

B. **Characteristic Profile:** Write a description of yourself as a health care worker that explains at least four (4) of the personal characteristics without using the actual words. A sentence describing empathy is shown as an example.

As a health care worker, I must have a sincere interest in people, and I must be able to identify with and understand another person's feelings, situation, and motives.

C. **Completion and Short Answer:** In the space provided, print the answer to the question or complete the statement.

1. List five (5) factors that contribute to good health and briefly describe why each factor is important.

2. Identify three (3) basic rules for the appearance of uniforms.

3. List three (3) basic rules to observe in regard to shoes worn in a health career.

4. List three (3) ways to control body odor.

5. List two (2) reasons why the nails must be kept short and clean.

6. Why is it important to keep long hair pinned back and off the collar when a job requires close patient contact?

7. What jewelry can be worn with a uniform?

8. What is the purpose of makeup?

9. What is wrong with the following statements or situations as they pertain to patients?
   a. "I think your problem is cholelithiasis."

   b. Radio playing loudly while preoperative care is discussed

   c. "I don't got any appointments at that time."

10. Define *listening*.

11. Nonverbal communication involves the use of _____, _____, _____, _____, and _____ to convey messages or ideas.

12. List three (3) common causes of communication barriers.

13. Identify two (2) ways to improve communications with a person who is blind or visually impaired.

14. Identify three (3) main barriers created by cultural diversity.

15. List four (4) senses a health care worker can use to make observations.

16. What is the difference between subjective and objective observations?

17. How should an error on a health care record be corrected?

18. Define *teamwork*.

19. List four (4) ways to develop good interpersonal relationships.

20. Briefly describe the characteristics of each of the following types of leaders:
    a. democratic:

    b. laissez-faire:

    c. autocratic:

21. Define *stress*.

22. List the four (4) steps that should be followed when a stressor causes a physical reaction in the body.

23. Identify a situation that always leads to stress in your life. Briefly describe how you can adapt to or deal with the situation to decrease or eliminate stress.

24. Explain the difference between short-term and long-term goals.

25. List the seven (7) steps of an effective time management plan.

CHAPTER 3 INTERNET SEARCHES

Use the suggested search engines in Chapter 9:4 of the textbook to search the Internet for additional information on the following topics:

1. *Uniform companies:* Search "uniform suppliers" to locate companies that sell professional uniforms and compare styles, prices, and so forth.

2. *Professional characteristics:* Choose a specific health care career and search for career descriptions; list the personal qualities or characteristics necessary for the career you have chosen.

3. *Communication:* Search for information on listening skills, nonverbal communication, and the communication process.

4. *Leadership:* Search for information on types and characteristics of leaders; evaluate which types would be most effective in guiding a health care team.

5. *Stress:* Search for information on stress and stress-reducing techniques.

6. *Time management:* Search for information on time management.

4:1 CAREERS IN HEALTH CARE

ASSIGNMENT SHEET

Grade _____ Name _____

INTRODUCTION: An individual who wants to work in health care has a wide variety of career choices. This assignment will help you review some of the careers.

INSTRUCTIONS: Read the information on Careers in Health Care. Then follow the instructions by each section to complete this assignment.

A. Health Career Search: All the careers listed are hidden in the following word search puzzle. Locate and circle the careers.

athletic trainer
biomedical equipment
dental hygienist
dietitian
electrocardiograph
electroencephalographic
geriatric aide

home health care
licensed practical nurse
medical laboratory
music therapist
nurse
occupational therapist
optometrist

paramedic
perfusionist
pharmacist
physical therapist
physician
psychologist
radiologic technologist

recreational therapist
respiratory therapy
social worker
surgical technician
veterinarian

```
M L O O K O I B T M U S I C T H E R A P I S T A E G C
E A D R P Z U I H E L P G N S R A D I P E R S F L E R
D I E E A H O O D E N G R A F I N D W O R D I C E S T
I D N K R S T M T O R T S I R T E M O T P O G Y C T P
C E T R A V H E F E D I A C I R T A I R E G O S T O H
A R A O T E I D L A N T N I L A H P E C A R L O R R Y
L A L W H T S I W A T S I N O I S U F R E P O H O E S
L C H L E E I C O S V E N H S T E C H N I C N R E N I
A H Y A R R S A P E T S I C A M R A H P O R H O N I C
B T G I M I L L O W O R K E R O T H E R A P C C C A A
O L I C E N S E D P R A C T I C A L N U R S E S E R L
R A E O F A S Q U H E C I L O A S S I S T A T N P T T
A E N S A R N U R Y O T L A N O I T A P U C C O H C H
T H I N K I L I M S S H O C E U R O F A T I I G A I E
O E S O C A A P Y I N E R I S T R A P E M S G C L T R
R M T R I N T M U C U R E G E R I S T S Q U O P O E A
Y O G D E I U E B I O A M R P H Y S E B E L L A G L P
R H E S T N E N M A S P M U S C I E I G Y H O M R H I
O M M L U P T T S N C I O S H P A R A M E D I C A T S
F P S Y C H O L O G I S T O N A I T I T E I D E P A T
R A D I O N T E L E C T R O C A R D I O G R A P H I N
E N T S I P A R E H T L A N O I T A E R C E R P I H O
P R E S P I R A T O R Y T H E R A P Y S R U N A C A L
```

B. Matching: Place the letter of the abbreviation in Column B in the space provided by the career it represents in Column A.

Column A	Column B
____ 1. Occupational Therapist	A. CBET
____ 2. Doctor of Dental Medicine	B. CLT
____ 3. Emergency Medical Technician	C. CMA
____ 4. Certified Biomedical Equipment Technician	D. DC
____ 5. Registered Nurse	E. DMD
____ 6. Registered Dietitian	F. DDS
____ 7. Doctor of Dental Surgery	G. DPM
____ 8. Doctor of Podiatric Medicine	H. DVM or VMD
____ 9. Certified Medical Assistant	I. ECG
____ 10. Electrocardiograph Technician	J. EEG
____ 11. Physical Therapist	K. EMT
____ 12. Doctor of Chiropractic	L. LPN or LVN
____ 13. Licensed Practical/Vocational Nurse	M. MD
____ 14. Doctor of Medicine	N. OT
____ 15. Certified Laboratory Technician	O. PT
____ 16. Veterinarian	P. RD
____ 17. Electroencelphalographic Technician	Q. RN
____ 18. Respiratory Therapist	R. RT

C. Completion or Short Answer: In the space provided, print the word(s) that best completes the statement or answers the question.

1. Briefly describe the educational requirements for the following degrees.

   Associate's:

   Bachelor's:

   Master's:

2. Identify the following methods used to ensure the skill and competency of health care workers:

   a. A professional association or government agency regulating a particular health career issues a statement that a person has fulfilled the requirements of education and performance and meets the standards and qualifications established:

   b. A government agency authorizes an individual to work in a given occupation after the individual has completed an approved education program and passed a state board test:

   c. A regulatory body in a health care area administers examinations and maintains a list of qualified personnel:

3. What is the difference between a technician and a technologist?

4. Who are multicompetent or multiskilled workers?

   Why do smaller facilities and rural areas hire these workers?

5. Define *entrepreneur*.

   List three (3) characteristics of a person who is an entrepreneur.

6. The following statements describe medical specialities (see Table 4-9). Print the correct name of the specialty or specialist in the space provided.

   a. _____ diseases and disorders of the eye

   b. _____ diseases and disorders of the mind

   c. _____ disorders of the brain and nervous system

   d. _____ diseases of the female reproductive system

   e. _____ diseases of the kidney, bladder, or urinary system

   f. _____ illness or injury in all age groups

   g. _____ diagnosis and treatment of tumors

7. The following statements describe health careers. Print the correct name of the career in the space provided.

   a. _____ work under supervision of a dentist to remove stains and deposits from the teeth, expose and develop X-rays

   b. _____ work with X-rays, radiation, nuclear medicine, ultrasound

   c. _____ provide basic care for medical emergencies, illness, injury

   d. _____ organize and code patient records, gather statistical data

   e. _____ nurse assistant who works with elderly individuals

   f. _____ dispense medications on written orders from others who are authorized to prescribe medications

   g. _____ use recreational and leisure activities as form of treatment

8. Review the different health careers and find at least two (2) careers that interest you. List the two careers and include a brief description of the duties and educational requirements of each. Also include a brief statement about why you might like to work in each career.

9. Choose one of the careers listed previously and write to an organization that will provide additional information about the career. Let your instructor check your letter before you mail it. Organizations and addresses are provided after each career cluster in the textbook. If you have access to the Internet, contact the organization by using the Internet address provided or by doing an Internet search. This will allow you to read or print a hard copy of information on the career.

4:2 Demonstrating Brushing and Flossing Techniques

Using correct brushing and flossing techniques is essential to prevent dental disease. Teaching the patient the correct methods to use is part of the responsibility of a dental assistant.

Correct brushing and flossing are important parts of prophylactic (preventive) care. Purposes include:

■ Prevention of decay, or **carious lesions** (**caries**).

■ Removal of plaque. **Plaque** is a thin, tenacious, filmlike deposit that adheres to the teeth and can lead to decay. It contains microorganisms and a protein substance.

■ Prevention of **halitosis** (bad breath).

The importance of proper brushing and flossing techniques must be stressed to the patient. Demonstrations should be given to all patients. Talk slowly and clearly. Repeat and stress important points.

The brushing technique taught will depend on the preference of the doctor. A common technique is the Bass method. The brush is placed at a 45° angle to the gumline and then a vibrating motion is used.

Five surfaces on each tooth must be cleaned:

■ *Chewing, or biting, surface*

■ *Facial surface:* the tooth side that faces the inside of the lips and cheeks; facial surfaces are seen from the front, as in a smile

■ *Lingual surface:* the tooth side nearest the tongue

■ *Side, or interproximal, surfaces:* the surfaces located between the teeth; there are two on each tooth; floss is used to clean these surfaces because a brush cannot get between the teeth

Toothbrushes vary in size, shape, and texture of the bristles. A soft-bristled brush is usually recommended. It will not injure the gum, or gingival tissue. The head of the brush should be the correct size and fit easily into the mouth. Brushes should be discarded when the bristles are frayed or worn. Many kinds of electric toothbrushes are also available. They are effective in cleaning the teeth if used correctly. They can be very beneficial for people with limited function of the hands and arms, such as people with arthritis.

Toothpastes or dentrifices are used to clean the teeth and provide a pleasant taste. Many doctors recommend toothpaste with fluoride. The American Dental Association supports the use of fluoride as an aid in preventing decay. Toothpastes with tartar control help prevent the hard deposits that accumulate on the teeth. Toothpastes with whitening agents help remove stains from teeth. The type of toothpaste recommended to the patient depends on the needs of the patient and the doctor's preference.

Dental floss is used to remove plaque and bacteria from the side surfaces of the teeth. Floss is available in waxed and unwaxed types. The type suggested to the patient depends on the doctor's preference. Both types are effective if used correctly.

STUDENT: *Complete the assignment sheet for 4:2, Demonstrating Brushing and Flossing Techniques. Then continue with the procedures.*

4:2 DEMONSTRATING BRUSHING AND FLOSSING TECHNIQUES

ASSIGNMENT SHEET

Grade _____ Name _____

INTRODUCTION: This assignment will help you review the main facts regarding brushing and flossing of the teeth.

INSTRUCTIONS: Review the information on Demonstrating Brushing and Flossing Techniques. In the space provided, print the word(s) that best completes the statement or answers the question.

1. List three (3) purposes or reasons for using correct brushing and flossing techniques.

2. Demonstrations on brushing and flossing should be given to _____. Talk _____ and _____. _____ and _____ important parts.

3. When the Bass technique for brushing is used, the brush is placed at _____ and then a _____ motion is used.

4. List the five (5) surfaces that must be cleaned on each tooth.

5. Which surfaces are not cleaned by brushing but are cleaned by flossing?

6. Which type of toothbrush is recommended in most cases? Why?

7. When should brushes be discarded?

8. What is the purpose of toothpaste or dentifrices?

9. Why is fluoride added to toothpaste?

10. List two (2) types of dental floss.

    Which type of floss should patients use?

Equipment and Supplies

Soft-textured toothbrush, demonstration model of teeth

Procedure

1. Assemble equipment.

2. Wash hands.

3. Introduce yourself. Identify the patient.

4. Explain the importance of correctly brushing the teeth. Stress that proper brushing helps prevent decay and removes plaque, a soft deposit leading to decay. Also stress that teeth should be brushed immediately after eating.

5. Suggest the use of a soft-textured brush to prevent gum damage.
   NOTE: If the doctor has recommended another type of toothbrush, follow the doctor's preference.

6. Use a toothbrush and demonstration model of teeth to show the patient how to brush the teeth.

7. Tell the patient to begin brushing in one area of the mouth and then to systematically brush each tooth. Suggest starting on the facial surfaces of the right, rear teeth.

8. Place the brush at a 45° angle to the gumline.

9. Rotate the brush slightly and gently push the bristles between the teeth.

10. Use a very short, back-and-forth, vibrating movement to clean the teeth.

11. Move the brush to the next group of teeth. Repeat steps 8 to 10. Continue until the facial surfaces of all the teeth are clean.

12. Repeat steps 8 to 10 on the lingual, or tongue, surfaces of the teeth. To brush the lingual surfaces of the front, or anterior, teeth, place the brush in a vertical position.

13. Brush the biting surfaces of all teeth. Place the brush on the surfaces. Use a very short, vibrating motion. Move the brush to the next area. Repeat until all biting surfaces are clean.

14. Stress to the patient that the areas between the teeth must be cleaned with floss.

15. Ask whether the patient has any questions. Make sure the patient understands the technique to use.
    NOTE: Asking the patient to demonstrate the technique is a good method of determining whether the main points have been understood.

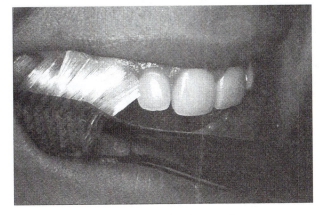

Place the brush at a 45° angle to the gumline.

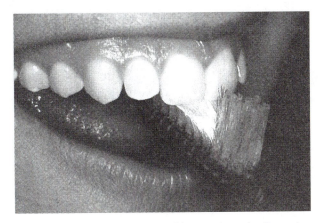

Hold the brush in a vertical position to clean the lingual, or tongue, surfaces of the anterior teeth.

Procedure 4:2A (cont.)

16. Clean and replace all equipment.

17. Wash hands.

Practice *Use the evaluation sheet for 4:2A, Demonstrating Brushing Technique, to practice this procedure. When you feel you have mastered this skill, sign the sheet and give it to your instructor for further action.*

✔**Final Checkpoint** Using the criteria listed on the evaluation sheet, your instructor will grade your performance.

Name _____ Date _____

Evaluated by _____

DIRECTIONS: Practice demonstrating brushing techniques according to the criteria listed. When you are ready for your final check, give this sheet to your instructor.

Demonstrating Brushing Techniques	Points Possible	Yes	No	Points Earned	Comments
1. Assembles equipment and supplies	4				
2. Washes hands	4				
3. Introduces self and identifies patient	4				
4. Stresses importance of brushing	8				
5. Uses soft-textured brush	8				
6. Suggests systematic method for brushing	8				
7. Places brush at 45-degree angle at gumline	8				
8. Rotates brush gently to get bristles in place	8				
9. Vibrates with short back-and-forth motion to clean tooth	8				
10. Cleans facial (front) surface	5				
11. Cleans lingual (tongue) surface	5				
12. Places brush vertically to do lingual (tongue) surface of front teeth	5				
13. Cleans biting surface	5				
14. Uses very short vibrating motion on biting surface	6				
15. Makes sure that patient understands method	6				
16. Replaces equipment	4				
17. Washes hands	4				
Totals	100				

Equipment and Supplies

Dental floss, demonstration model of teeth

Procedure

1. Assemble equipment.
2. Wash hands.
3. Introduce yourself. Identify the patient.
4. 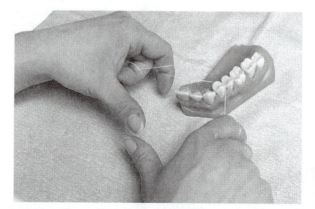Explain the importance of flossing. Stress that flossing is the way to remove food and plaque from between the teeth. Mention that this is an area where decay often begins.
5. Use dental floss and a demonstration model of the teeth to show the patient how to floss the teeth.
6. Remove 12 to 18 inches of floss from the spool.
   NOTE: Floss is waxed or unwaxed. The type recommended depends on the doctor's preference.
7. Wrap the floss around the middle fingers of both hands. This anchors the floss. As floss is used, unroll new floss from the middle finger of one hand and wrap used floss around the middle finger of the opposite hand.
8. To clean the upper (maxillary) teeth, wrap the floss around the index finger of one hand and the thumb of the other hand or the two thumbs. To clean the lower (mandibular) teeth, use the index fingers of both hands.
   NOTE: Floss still remains anchored on middle fingers.
9. Keep the fingers and thumb approximately 1 to 2 inches apart. This is the length of floss to be used.
10. Gently insert the floss between the teeth. Do not snap the floss into the gums.
    CAUTION: Snapping the floss into the gums can injure the gum tissue.
11. Gently slide the floss into the space between the gum and tooth. Stop when you feel resistance. Curve the floss into a C shape around the side of the tooth.
12. Hold the floss tightly against the tooth and move the floss away from the gum by scraping the floss up and down against the side of the tooth.
    CAUTION: A side-to-side or front-to-back motion could cut the gums.
13. Repeat steps 10 to 12 until both sides of every tooth in the mouth have been flossed. Move the floss on the fingers as it becomes soiled. Use fresh floss at all times.
14. Warn the patient that some bleeding and soreness may occur the first few times teeth are flossed. If bleeding or soreness continues, flossing should be stopped and the doctor notified.
15. Make sure the patient understands the procedure.
    NOTE: Asking the patient to demonstrate the technique is a good way to determine whether the main points have been understood.
16. Clean and replace all equipment.
17. Wash hands.

Practice *Use the evaluation sheet for 4:2B, Demonstrating Flossing Technique, to practice this procedure. When you feel you have mastered this skill, sign the sheet and give it to your instructor for further action.*

✔ **Final Checkpoint** Using the criteria listed on the evaluation sheet, your instructor will grade your performance.

After curving the floss into a C shape around the side of the tooth, use an up-and-down motion to clean the side.

4:2B EVALUATION SHEET

Name _____ Date _____

Evaluated by _____

DIRECTIONS: Practice demonstrating flossing techniques according to the criteria listed. When you are ready for your final check, give this sheet to your instructor.

Demonstrating Flossing Techniques	Points Possible	Yes	No	Points Earned	Comments
1. Assembles equipment and supplies	3				
2. Washes hands	3				
3. Introduces self and identifies patient	3				
4. Stresses importance of flossing	7				
5. Uses 12–18 inches of floss	6				
6. Anchors floss on middle fingers	6				
7. Wraps floss around index fingers and/or thumb or the two thumbs	6				
8. Leaves 1 to 2 inches of floss between fingers	6				
9. Inserts floss gently into space between gum and tooth	7				
10. Stresses not to snap floss in place	7				
11. Forms C around side of tooth	6				
12. Holds floss firmly by tooth and uses up-and-down motion	7				
13. Cleans both sides of every tooth	7				
14. Warns patient about bleeding or soreness	6				
15. Tells patient to call doctor if bleeding persists	6				
16. Makes sure that patient understands procedure	8				
17. Replaces equipment	3				
18. Washes hands	3				
Totals	100				

4:3 OPERATING THE MICROSCOPE

The **microscope** is a valuable tool used in many health professions. In order to obtain the desired results when working with the microscope, it is important that you first become familiar with its parts and how to use them correctly.

Many models of microscopes are available. A *monocular microscope* has one eyepiece, and a *binocular microscope* has two eyepieces. The quality of microscopes also varies, according to the type of lenses, attachments, and magnification ability. The compound, bright-field microscope, described in this unit, is one of the most commonly used microscopes. An epifluorescence microscope is used to detect antibodies and specific organisms by using a fluorescent dye stain. An electron microscope, which is extremely expensive and requires special expertise to operate, uses electron beams instead of a light source to view objects. Electron microscopes are used to view extremely small objects such as cell organelles and viruses. How-ever, all microscopes have one basic purpose. They are designed to magnify or enlarge objects so the objects become more visible.

Most microscopes contain the same basic parts. A list and a brief description of the function of each part follows. Parts are shown in the following figure.

- *Base:* The solid stand on which the microscope rests.

- *Arm:* The long, back stem of the microscope. In most cases the arm is used to carry the microscope.

- *Eyepiece(s):* The part(s) of the microscope through which the eye views the object or slide. The eyepiece usually has a magnification power of 10× (ten times). This means that it makes the object on the slide appear 10 times larger than normal. Some microscopes have zoom lenses. On these, the magnification can range from

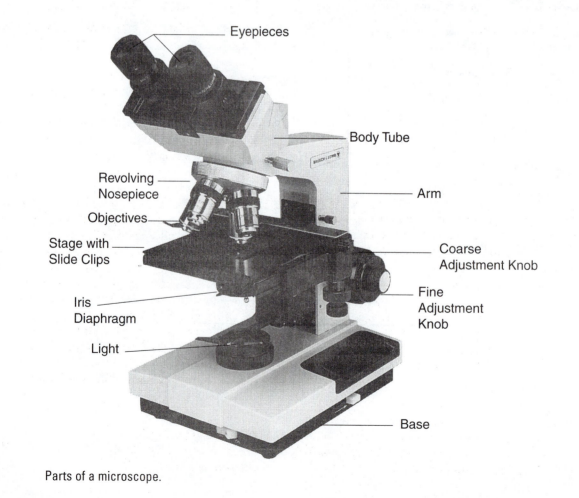

Parts of a microscope.

10× to 20×, depending on how the eyepiece is positioned. Special lens paper should be used to clean the eyepiece to avoid scratching the lenses. The eyepiece is also called the *ocular viewpiece.*

- *Objectives:* The parts of the microscope that magnify the object being viewed. They work with the eyepiece. A microscope may have three or four objectives, and they can vary. Some of the more common objectives are:

  (1) The low-power objective is the shortest in length. It magnifies the object being viewed four times (4×).

  (2) Another low-power objective magnifies the object 10 times (10×).

  (3) The high-power objectives magnify the object 40 or 45 times (40× or 45×).

  (4) The oil-immersion (OI) objective usually has a magnification power of 95× to 100×. Oil must be used with this objective because the image is usually too dark to be seen otherwise. The oil concentrates the light. A drop of immersion oil is placed on the slide. The oil-immersion objective is carefully rotated into the drop of oil. Care must be taken to prevent the oil from coming into contact with any of the other objectives on the microscope.

  NOTE: Smaller specimens require greater magnification. However, the high-power objectives have small openings. Therefore, to view small specimens, use a high-power objective and more light. For large specimens, use low-power objectives and less light. Special lens paper should be used to clean the objectives.

- *Revolving nosepiece:* The section to which the objectives are attached. It is turned to change the objective being used.

- *Stage:* The flat platform for the slide. Slide clips are located on the stage to hold the slide in place.

- *Coarse adjustment:* The larger knob on the arm. It moves the objectives up and down and also brings the slide into rough focus. The coarse adjustment should be used only on the low power (10×) objective. It is important to watch the stage while moving the objectives to avoid breaking the slide and/or objectives.

- *Fine adjustment:* The smaller knob on the arm. It moves the objectives slowly for a precise and clear image. The fine adjustment is used on the low-power (10×), high-power (40–45×), and oil immersion (95–100×) objectives.

- *Iris diaphragm:* A circular structure directly underneath the stage. The diaphragm controls the amount of light that enters the microscope through the bottom of the stage. To increase or decrease the amount of light, turn the diaphragm to a larger or smaller hole.

- *Illuminating light:* Located under the stage, the illuminating light provides the necessary light for viewing; the amount of light is controlled by the iris diaphragm.

- *Body tube:* The section that connects the eyepiece and the objectives.

To determine total magnification of an object (how many times you are magnifying or enlarging the object) multiply the power of the eyepiece times the power of the objective in use.

- *Example 1:* If the eyepiece is 10× and the objective is 4×, multiply the 10 and the 4.

$$10 \times 4 = 40$$

  The object is magnified or enlarged 40 times its original size.

- *Example 2:* Eyepiece is 20×, and objective is 40X.

$$20 \times 40 = 800$$

  You are enlarging the object 800 times.

Proper care and cleaning of any microscope is important because dirt and dust can interfere with proper viewing and damage the delicate glass on the eyepiece and objectives. The glass in the eyepiece and objectives should be cleaned with special lens paper. Paper towels, tissues, and cloths can scratch the delicate glass. The rest of the microscope should be wiped clean with a damp, soft cloth after use. When oil is used with an oil-immersion objective, the oil should be wiped off immediately after use because it can seep into the lens case. Before the microscope is stored, the low-power objective should be in place. The nosepiece should be moved to its lowest position. When the microscope is not in use, it should be covered with a dust cover or stored in a dust-free cabinet. It is also important to avoid jarring or bumping the microscope because it is a delicate instrument. To carry or move a microscope, place one hand firmly on the arm and the other hand under the base. Always put the microscope down gently when placing it on a desk or counter. Before using any microscope, read and follow the specific operating instructions provided by the manufacturer.

STUDENT: *Complete the assignment sheet for 4:3, Operating the Microscope. Then continue with the procedure.*

4:3 OPERATING THE MICROSCOPE

ASSIGNMENT SHEET

Grade _____ Name _____

INTRODUCTION: This assignment will help you understand the parts of the microscope and basic operating principles.

INSTRUCTIONS: Review the information on Operating the Microscope. In the space provided, print the word(s) that best completes the statement or answers the question. Identify the parts of the microscope, and write their names beside the corresponding number in the column.

1.

2.

3.

4.

5.

6.

7.

8.

9.

10.

11.

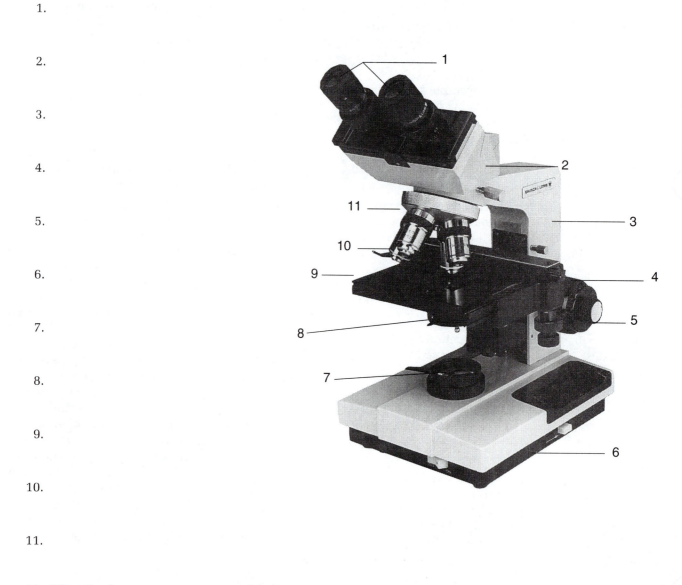

12. What do electron microscopes use to view objects?

13. Why is an epifluorescence microscope used?

14. What might happen if you lower the objective with the coarse adjustment while looking through the eyepiece?

15. How do you increase the amount of light that enters the microscope through the hole in the stage?

16. Why must you use special lens paper to clean the eyepiece and the objectives?

17. What is the function (use of) the coarse adjustment knob?

18. What is the function of the fine adjustment knob?

19. What is an oil-immersion objective used for?

20. If the eyepiece you are using has a magnification power of 10×, what will the total magnification be with the following objectives? (How much would you enlarge each object?)
    a. 4×
    b. 10×
    c. 40×

21. If the eyepiece you are using is 20×, what will the total magnification be with the following objectives?
    a. 4×
    b. 10×
    c. 40×

22. How should a microscope be stored?

Equipment and Supplies

Microscope; lens paper; slide and cover slip; hair, paper, or other small object; drop of water; immersion oil

Procedure

1. Assemble equipment.

2. Wash hands.

   ⚠ **CAUTION:** Wear gloves and observe standard precautions while handling any specimen contaminated by blood or body fluids, or while examining pathogenic organisms.

3. Use a prepared slide or get a clean slide. Place a human hair, shred of paper, or other small object on the slide. Add a drop of water or normal saline. Cover with a clean cover slip by holding the cover slip at an angle and allowing it to drop on the specimen.

   NOTE: Make sure there are no air bubbles between the slide and cover slip. If air bubbles are present, remove the cover slip and position it again.

4. Use lens paper to clean the eyepiece (ocular viewpiece) and the objectives.

   ⚠ **CAUTION:** Do not use any other material to clean these surfaces. Towels, rags, and tissues can scratch these surfaces.

5. Turn on the illuminating light. Open the iris diaphragm so that the largest hole is located directly under the hole in the stage platform.

6. Turn the revolving nosepiece until the low-power objective clicks into place.

7. Place the slide on the stage. Fasten it with the slide clips.

   NOTE: Avoid getting fingerprints or smudges on the slide.

8. Watch the stage and slide. Turn the coarse adjustment so that the objective moves down close to the slide.

   ⚠ **CAUTION:** Do *not* look into the eyepiece while moving the objective down. The objective could crack the slide and/or be damaged.

9. Now, look through the eyepiece. Slowly turn the body tube upward until the object comes into focus.

10. Change to the fine adjustment. Turn the knob slowly until the object comes into its sharpest focus.

11. Do the following while still using low power:

    a. Move the slide to the right while looking through the eyepiece. In which direction does the image move?

    b. Move the slide to the left. In which direction does the image move?

    c. Move the iris diaphragm to change the amount of light. How does this affect the image?

12. Without moving the body tube, turn the revolving nosepiece until the high-power objective is in place. Focus with the fine adjustment only.

    ⚠ **CAUTION:** Watch the slide while turning the objectives to avoid breaking the slide or objectives.

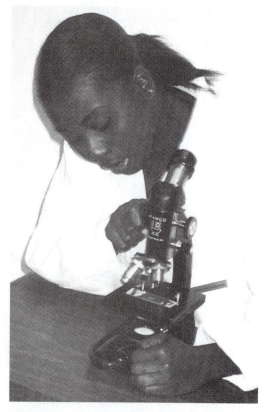

Watch the stage and slide while using the coarse adjustment to move the objective downward.

Procedure 4:3 (cont.)

13. Under high power, make the following observations:

   a. How does the amount of light compare with that needed under low power? (You may need to adjust the diaphragm for better viewing.)

   b. Do you see a larger or a smaller area of the object than was seen under low power?

14. If the microscope has an oil-immersion objective, do the following:

   a. Turn the revolving nosepiece until the oil-immersion objective is in position. Focus with fine adjustment only.

   CAUTION: Watch the slide while turning the objectives to avoid breaking the slide or objectives.

   b. Move the oil-immersion objective slightly to either side so that no objective is in position.

   c. Place a small drop of immersion oil on the part of the slide that will be directly under the objective.

   CAUTION: Use the oil sparingly.

   d. Move the oil-immersion objective back into position, taking care that no other objective comes into contact with the oil. Make sure that the oil-immersion objective is touching the drop of oil.

   e. Look through the eyepiece and use the fine adjustment to bring the slide into focus.

   f. Move the diaphragm as necessary to adjust the amount of light for viewing the slide.

   g. When you are done viewing the slide, turn the revolving nosepiece until the low-power objective is in position.

   CAUTION: Make sure no other objective comes into contact with the oil on the slide.

   h. Use lens paper to carefully remove all the oil from the oil-immersion objective.

15. When you are done viewing the slide, remove the slide and the cover slip. Wash and dry both items.

   CAUTION: Handle both with care. They break easily.

16. Use the special lens paper to clean the eyepiece and the objectives.

   CAUTION: Do *not* use any other material to clean these parts. Towels, rags, and tissues can scratch these surfaces.

17. Use a damp, soft cloth to wipe the other parts of the microscope.

18. Using the coarse adjustment, move the low-power objective so that it is in its lowest position, down close to the stage.

19. Turn off the illuminating light.

20. Place the cover back on the microscope. This protects it from dust in the room. The microscope can also be stored in a dust-free cabinet.

   CAUTION: Remember to place one hand on the arm and the other hand under the base while moving the microscope.

21. Make sure that the microscope is kept away from the counter's edge. This prevents the microscope from being knocked to the floor.

22. Clean and replace all equipment.

23. Remove gloves. Wash hands.

Practice *Use the evaluation sheet for 4:3, Operating the Microscope, to practice this procedure. When you feel you have mastered this skill, sign the sheet and give it to your instructor for further action.*

✔ **Final Checkpoint** Using the criteria listed on the evaluation sheet, your instructor will grade your performance.

Name _____ Date _____

Evaluated by _____

DIRECTIONS: Practice operating the microscope according to the criteria listed. When you are ready for your final check, give this sheet to your instructor.

Operating the Microscope	Points Possible	Yes	No	Points Earned	Comments
1. Assembles equipment and supplies	2				
2. Washes hands and puts on gloves if needed	2				
3. Identifies parts:					
Arm	2				
Base	2				
Stage	2				
Eyepiece	2				
Revolving nosepiece	2				
Objectives	2				
Light	2				
Iris diaphragm	2				
Slide clips	2				
Coarse adjustment	2				
Fine adjustment	2				
Body tube	2				
4. Cleans slide and cover slip	3				
5. Places specimen on slide	3				
6. Adds drop of water or normal saline to slide	3				
7. Adds cover slip without air bubbles	3				
8. Positions low objective	3				
9. Turns on illuminating light	3				
10. Anchors slide on stage with slide clips	3				
11. Lowers objective while watching slide	3				
12. Uses coarse adjustment for rough focus	3				
13. Uses fine adjustment for precise focus	3				
14. Increases or decreases amount of light as needed by turning iris diaphragm	3				
15. Switches to high power	3				
16. Focuses with fine adjustment	3				

Evaluation 4:3 (cont.)

Operating the Microscope	Points Possible	Yes	No	Points Earned	Comments
17. Uses oil-immersion objective:					
Positions oil-immersion objective	2				
Focuses with fine adjustment	2				
Moves objective to side	2				
Puts small drop of oil on slide	2				
Repositions objective in oil	2				
Focuses with fine adjustment	2				
Cleans objective with lens paper when done	2				
18. Cleans slide and cover slip thoroughly	3				
19. Cleans eyepiece(s) and objectives with lens paper	3				
20. Lowers low power objective to stage	3				
21. Turns off light	3				
22. Covers for storage	3				
23. Cleans and replaces all equipment	2				
24. Removes gloves if worn and washes hands	2				
Totals	100				

This section provides facts about administering oxygen. *Check your legal responsibilities with regard to this procedure.* Some states prohibit administration of oxygen by a health care assistant.

The blood must have oxygen. The blood's supply of oxygen is normally obtained from the air. Air is approximately 20 percent oxygen. As a result of accident, injury, or respiratory disease, however, the body may be unable to take in enough oxygen or to use oxygen effectively. In such cases, oxygen can be given to the patient by various means.

The signs of an oxygen shortage are rapid and shallow respirations, rapid pulse, restlessness, and cyanosis. A deficiency of oxygen is called *hypoxia*. Lack of oxygen can cause brain damage in 4 to 6 minutes.

A physician's order is usually required for the administration of oxygen. The order will include the method of administration and the concentration to be given. In cases of extreme emergency, oxygen can be started with standard concentrations, and the physician notified as soon as possible. Most rescue teams, ambulance personnel, and others involved in emergency work follow specific orders regarding oxygen administration.

Oxygen is usually administered by one of the following methods:

■ *Mask:* The mask should cover the mouth and the nose. It should fit snugly to prevent loss of oxygen, but it should not be so tight as to cause discomfort to the patient. Oxygen by mask is the method of administration used most frequently by rescue personnel. It provides the highest concentration of oxygen. However, some patients are frightened by the mask. A careful explanation of its purpose along with constant reassurance are necessary. The rate of flow by mask is usually 6 to 10 liters per minute.

■ *Cannula:* The cannula consists of two small, curved, plastic tubes, which are placed one in each nostril. The other end of the cannula is attached to an oxygen tank or unit. The patient must be instructed to breathe through the nose. If the patient opens the mouth to breathe, the concentration of oxygen is reduced. The rate of flow by cannula is usually 2 to 6 liters per minute.

■ *Catheter:* The catheter is a long, narrow, plastic or rubber tube that is passed through a nostril and to the throat. It is inserted by a physician, registered nurse, respiratory therapist, or other specially trained individual. The rate of flow is usually 2 to 6 liters per minute.

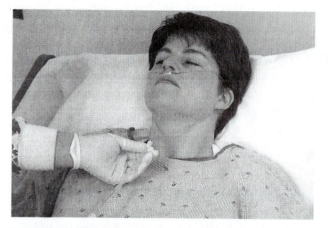

When a nasal cannula is used to provide oxygen, the patient must breathe through the nose.

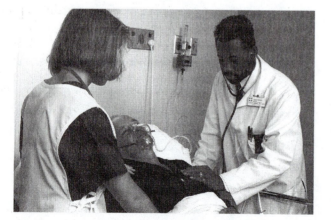

The oxygen mask covers the nose and mouth and provides a high concentration of oxygen.

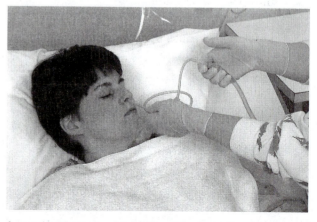

A nasal catheter is passed through a nostril and to the pharynx, or throat, to administer oxygen.

- *Tent:* The tent surrounds the patient with a high concentration of oxygen. It is often used for small children or restless patients who are not able to cooperate well with other methods. Oxygen and humidity are provided. A common example is a croupette used with infants and small children. The flow rate is usually 10 to 12 liters per minute.

Pure oxygen is very drying and can damage or irritate mucous membranes. Therefore, oxygen must be moisturized by passing it through water before it is administered to the patient. A humidifier is used to moisturize oxygen. The humidifier must be filled with distilled water to the proper level, usually one-half to two-thirds of the container. Most humidifiers are marked for the proper level. Distilled water is usually used to prevent mineral deposits on the equipment. In emergency situations when oxygen is given for short periods of time during transportation to a medical facility, the oxygen may not be humidified.

Safety precautions must be observed when oxygen is in use. Although oxygen does not explode, burning is more rapid and intense in the presence of oxygen. Flammable materials (those that burn) will burn much more rapidly in the presence of oxygen. The following precautions should be taken whenever oxygen is in use:

- Smoking, lighting cigarettes or matches, burning candles, and the use of open flames are prohibited when oxygen is in use. In patient-care areas, a warning sign reading, for example, "No Smoking—Oxygen" is placed on the door to the patient's room, on the bed, or on the wall nearby. Warning labels are also sometimes placed on tanks used by emergency rescue personnel.

- The sign is not enough. The patient must be cautioned against smoking. Observers at the scene of an accident or emergency situation and visitors in a patient-care area must also be told to avoid smoking.

- The use of electrically operated equipment, which could cause sparks, should be avoided.

- Never use flammable liquids such as nail polish remover or adhesive tape remover.

- Cotton blankets should be used in place of wool or nylon. In addition, all bed linen, bedspreads, and gowns or pajamas should be cotton instead of synthetic materials. Cotton is static-free, and its use decreases the danger of static electricity.

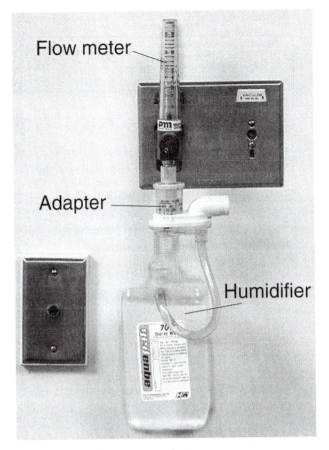

A humidifier is used to moisturize oxygen.

- Frequent inspections must be made of any area where oxygen is in use. Sources of sparks or static electricity should be removed.

A patient who is receiving oxygen must be checked frequently. Quality of respirations should be noted. Mouth and nose care must be provided if a mask, catheter, or cannula is used. The rate of flow of oxygen should be checked. Watch to make sure that the patient and/or visitors do *not* change the liter flow. If a humidifier is used, water (preferably distilled) must be added to the humidifier as needed. Safety precautions should be checked. In many facilities, oxygen administration is the responsibility of the respiratory therapy department. However, the health care worker, who is with the patient more frequently, should always be aware of safety precautions and check patients carefully. Any abnormal observations should be reported immediately.

STUDENT: *Complete the assignment sheet for 4:4, Administering Oxygen. Then continue with the procedure.*

4:4 ADMINISTERING OXYGEN

ASSIGNMENT SHEET

Grade _____ Name _____

INTRODUCTION: The following assignment will help you learn the main points of oxygen administration.

INSTRUCTIONS: Review the information on Administering Oxygen. Then print the word(s) that best completes the statement or answers the question.

1. Why is it important to check your legal responsibilities before administering oxygen?

2. Define *hypoxia*.

3. List three (3) signs of oxygen shortage.

4. List the four (4) main methods of administering oxygen. Then list the usual flow rate for each method.

   Method   *Flow Rate*

5. Why is oxygen usually passed through water before being administered to a patient?

6. Why is distilled water used in the oxygen humidifier?

7. List three (3) safety rules that must be observed when oxygen is in use.

8. A patient who is receiving oxygen must be checked frequently. List three (3) special checkpoints that must be observed.

9. Who is usually responsible for oxygen administration in health care facilities?

Equipment and Supplies

Oxygen mask, cannula, or tent; tubing and gauge; oxygen tank or supply; distilled water (if humidifier is used); pen or pencil

CAUTION: Some states prohibit the administration of oxygen by a health care assistant. Check your legal responsibilities in regard to this procedure.

Procedure

1. Read the physician's orders or obtain orders from your immediate supervisor. In emergency rescue situations, standard orders are usually provided for victims requiring oxygen. The orders should state the method of administration and liter flow per minute.

2. Assemble equipment.

3. Knock on the door and pause before entering. Introduce yourself. Identify the patient. Explain the procedure to the patient. Patients are often apprehensive. Reassure as needed.

4. Wash hands. In emergency situations, this may not be possible.

5. Connect the tubing from the oxygen supply (tank or wall unit) to the tubing on the mask or cannula. If a humidifier is used, check the water level to make sure the water supply is adequate.

   NOTE: Fill the container with distilled water, if needed. Distilled water prevents mineral deposits from forming.

6. Turn on the oxygen supply.

   CAUTION: Do not insert the nasal cannula or apply the mask at this time. Regulate the gauge to the correct liter flow rate per minute.

   CAUTION: Make sure to follow specific manufacturer's instructions or agency policy for connecting and turning on the oxygen supply. Do *not* operate any oxygen equipment until you have been specifically instructed on how to use it.

7. Check to be sure that oxygen is passing through the tubing. Place your hand by the outlet on the mask or cannula.

8. Put on disposable gloves.

   CAUTION: Observe all standard precautions if contact with the patient's oral or nasal secretions is possible.

9. With the oxygen still flowing, apply the mask or cannula to the patient. If a mask is used, position it over the patient's nose and mouth. Adjust the strap so that it fits snugly but does not apply pressure to the face. If a cannula is used, place the two tips in the patient's nostrils and loop the tubing around each ear. Adjust the straps at the neck so that the tips remain in position. Instruct the patient to breathe through the nose.

10. If a tent is used, it is first filled with oxygen; then, the prescribed liter flow is set. The humidifier is filled to the marked level with distilled water. The tent is placed over the bed or crib, and the edges are tucked in on all sides to prevent oxygen loss. A cotton blanket, bath blanket, or sheet can be used to provide a cuff around the loose end covering the patient.

11. Check the surrounding area to make sure all safety precautions are being observed. Eliminate any sources of sparks or flames. Caution any visitors and the patient against smoking while the oxygen is in use. In a patient-care area, make sure a sign is posted on the door or in the immediate area.

12. Check the patient at frequent intervals.
    - Note respirations, color, restlessness, or discomfort.
    - Provide skin care to the face and/or nose, if a mask or cannula is used.
    - Check the skin behind the ears and provide skin care if a nasal cannula is used.

Procedure 4:4 (cont.)

- At times, it may be necessary to use a towel or cloth to dry the inside of the mask, because moisture will accumulate in the mask.
- If a nasal cannula is used, check the tips to make sure they are open and not plugged by mucus.
- Provide oral hygiene frequently.
- Check the water level, if a humidifier is used.
- Check the gauge and make sure the liter flow rate is correct.
- Report any abnormal conditions immediately.

13. When the oxygen is discontinued, make sure that the oxygen supply is turned off. Follow specific manufacturer's instructions or agency policy. Clean and replace all equipment. Most masks and cannulas are disposable and are discarded after use. If the items are not disposable, they should be cleaned and disinfected according to established agency policy.

14. Wash hands.

15. Report and/or record all required information on the patient's chart or the agency form, for example, date; time; oxygen per mask at 6 L/min, R 16 deep and even; and your signature and title. Report any unusual observations immediately.

Practice *Use the evaluation sheet for 4:4, Administering Oxygen, to practice this procedure. When you feel you have mastered this skill, sign the sheet and give it to your instructor for further action.*

✔ **Final Checkpoint** Using the criteria listed on the evaluation sheet, your instructor will grade your performance.

Name _____ Date _____

Evaluated by _____

DIRECTIONS: Practice administering oxygen according to the criteria listed. When you are ready for your final check, give this sheet to your instructor.

Administering Oxygen	Points Possible	Yes	No	Points Earned	Comments
1. Checks doctor's order or obtains orders from immediate supervisor	4				
2. Assembles equipment and supplies	3				
3. Knocks on door, introduces self, and identifies patient	3				
4. Explains procedure to patient and reassures as needed	3				
5. Washes hands	3				
6. Connects tubing to mask/cannula	4				
7. Checks water supply if humidifier used and adds distilled water as needed	4				
8. Turns on oxygen supply	4				
9. Regulates gauge for ordered liter flow or sets as follows if no specific order:					
Mask: 6–10 liters	2				
Cannula: 2–6 liters	2				
Catheter: 2–6 liters	2				
Tent: 10–12 liters	2				
10. Checks for oxygen flow by placing hand at outlet	4				
11. Puts on gloves	4				
12. Applies mask:					
Positions over mouth and nose	3				
Adjusts strap until snug	3				
13. Applies nasal cannula:					
Places tips in nostrils	3				
Adjusts straps so position of tips maintained	3				
Instructs patient to breathe through nose	3				
14. Applies tent:					
Fills with oxygen	3				
Tucks in all edges	3				

Evaluation 4:4 (cont.)

Administering Oxygen	Points Possible	Yes	No	Points Earned	Comments
15. Checks area for all of the following safety precautions:					
Eliminates sources of sparks or flames	3				
Cautions everyone against smoking	3				
Posts sign in patient care area	3				
16. Checks patient and area frequently for following points:					
Respirations	2				
Color	2				
Restlessness/discomfort	2				
Provides skin care to face/nose/ears	2				
Checks water level if humidifier used	2				
Checks gauge for correct liter flow	2				
17. Reports any abnormal observations immediately	4				
18. Cleans and replaces all equipment after use	3				
19. Removes gloves and washes hands	3				
20. Records/reports all required information	4				
Totals	100				

4:5 COMPLETING A STATISTICAL DATA SHEET

Medical records vary, but some forms are used for certain purposes. Common forms are **statistical data** sheets or cards. All records are considered to be **confidential**. *No* information can be released from the records without the written consent of the patient. These forms belong to the physician or agency. They should be locked up when not in use.

Statistical data sheets are also called *registration forms*, *patient information forms*, or other similar names. This form is usually completed on a patient's first visit to an office or health agency. It contains basic reference information about the patient. The form may be a sheet of paper, an index card, or even the inside of the patient's folder. In many offices, the information is entered into a computer database. A sample entry screen is shown in the following figure. No matter what type of form is used, most contain the following information:

- patient's name in full
- patient's address, including city and zip code
- patient's telephone number
- patient's marital status, gender, and birthdate
- patient's place of employment
- name of the person responsible for the account
- insurance company information including address, policy and group numbers, and other pertinent information
- name of referring physician or other person

```
                                                    Screen ID # 5-1
ACCOUNT INFORMATION   Account Number _____
Last Name _____   First Name _____ M.I. ____
Address  _____   Social Security # ___-__-__
City     _____   State _____ Zip Code _____
Home Phone _____   Business Phone _____
Account Date __/__/__ Pri. Doctor __ Referring Doctor _____
Type Account ___ Fee Group ___   Number of Plans ___ Number of Dependents ___
Monthly Payment _____.00          Percentage of Discount __%

PERSONS COVERED BY ACCOUNT          FINANCIAL INFORMATION
Name                     S R Birth date
First Name   Last Name   E E MM/DD/YY   Balance        $ _____
                         X L            Date Last Pay    __/__/__
                                        Amount Last Pay $ _____
 _____   _____   __ __ __/__/__   Balance Current $ _____
 _____   _____   __ __ __/__/__   Balance 30 Day  $ _____
 _____   _____   __ __ __/__/__   Balance 60 Day  $ _____
 _____   _____   __ __ __/__/__   Balance 90 Day  $ _____
 _____   _____   __ __ __/__/__   Balance 120 Day $ _____

E - Edit, S - Save, A - Abandon, F - Finish, M - Account Message _____
F1-New F2-Daily F3-Report F4-Update F5-Post F6-Pull F7-Mail F8-Recall F9-Notes
```

Statistical data about the patient can be entered into a computer database by using a patient entry screen.

In most agencies this information is typed on the form or keyed into a computer database. If a computer is used, a printed copy may be placed in the patient's record. Care must be taken to ensure that all information is accurate. Double-check numbers and spelling.

In most agencies, the health care worker will complete the statistical data information. The physician or another authorized person will do all parts of the medical history.

The patient must have privacy when being questioned. A separate room should be used, and the door to the room should be closed. Specific questions must be asked. It is essential that questions be asked in a professional rather than prying manner. It is also important to make sure the patient understands the meaning of all questions. Information obtained must be accurate and complete. Facts should be rechecked as necessary. The patient should be given time to think about each question. It is important that the patient feels relaxed and at ease during the questioning. Note any additional information that the patient provides if it seems important. If no specific areas are provided on the forms for this type information, be sure the physician or other appropriate person is made aware of the information.

Legal requirements must be observed while working with medical records. It is essential to remember that all information on the record is confidential and cannot be given to any other individual, agency, or insurance company without the written permission of the patient. All records must be maintained for the period of time required by law. If an error is made while recording a medical record, the error should be crossed out in red ink, dated, and initialed. Correct information is then recorded.

An awareness of cultural diversity is essential when information is obtained. In some cultures, individuals feel it is disrespectful to speak of the dead. A patient may hesitate to discuss family history and illness if the person is deceased. A similar situation may exist in cases of adoption where biological family history is not known. An interpreter may be needed if a patient has limited English and speaks a foreign language. Patients may refuse to discuss family problems that may be causing stress and/or physical problems if they believe that this is personal information. If an individual has a cultural belief that illness is caused as a punishment for sin, the patient may not want to discuss specific symptoms or problems. In some cultures, individuals do not discuss pain. These individuals believe pain is something that must be tolerated and accepted; acknowledging pain is a sign of weakness. Many individuals may be hesitant to discuss cultural or religious remedies they have tried, such as herbal remedies, acupuncture, witchcraft, or religious rituals. The health care worker must show respect, tolerance, and acceptance of a patient's cultural and religious beliefs while obtaining information for the record.

The final version of the record is usually typed or keyed into a computer program and printed for the patient's permanent record. Make sure any handwritten copy is legible and clear. Double-check all information to make sure it has been recorded correctly.

Some common abbreviations used on medical records and forms are as follows:

- *S* for single
- *M* for married
- *W* for widowed
- *D* for divorced
- *O* for negative or none
- *l and w* for living and well
- *d* for died (year of death is usually placed after the symbol)
- *NA* or *N/A* for not applicable, or does not apply

STUDENT: *Complete the assignment sheet for 4:5, Completing a Statistical Data Sheet. Then continue with the procedure.*

4:5 COMPLETING A STATISTICAL DATA SHEET

ASSIGNMENT SHEET

Grade _____ Name _____

INTRODUCTION: This assignment sheet will help you review basic facts about statistical data sheets.

INSTRUCTIONS: Read the information on Completing a Statistical Data Sheet. In the space provided, print the word(s) that best completes the statement or answers the question.

1. List two (2) other names for statistical data sheets.

2. List five (5) kinds of information that are usually found on any statistical data sheet.

3. Information on medical records is _____ and should not be released without the _____ of the patient. The records should be _____ when not in use.

4. How can you provide privacy for the patient while obtaining information for the data form?

5. If a patient does not speak English, what must you do?

6. Print the meaning of the following symbols or abbreviations commonly found or used on medical records.

   a. S—   e. O—

   b. M—   f. l & w—

   c. W—   g. NA—

   d. D—   h. d—

STATISTICAL DATA SHEET

PATIENT INFORMATION

DATE:

PATIENT'S NAME	MARITAL STATUS					DATE OF BIRTH	SOCIAL SECURITY NO.
	S	M	W	DIV	SEP		

STREET ADDRESS ☐ PERMANENT ☐ TEMPORARY	CITY AND STATE		ZIP CODE	HOME PHONE NO.

PATIENT'S EMPLOYER	OCCUPATION (INDICATE IF STUDENT)	HOW LONG EMPLOYED?	BUSINESS PHONE NO.

EMPLOYER'S STREET ADDRESS	CITY AND STATE	ZIP CODE

IN CASE OF EMERGENCY CONTACT:	DRIVERS LIC. NO.

SPOUSE'S NAME

SPOUSE'S EMPLOYER	OCCUPATION (INDICATE IF STUDENT)	HOW LONG EMPLOYED?	BUSINESS PHONE NO.

EMPLOYER'S STREET ADDRESS	CITY AND STATE	ZIP CODE

WHO REFERRED YOU TO THIS PRACTICE?

IF THE PATIENT IS A MINOR OR STUDENT

MOTHER'S NAME	STREET ADDRESS, CITY, STATE AND ZIP CODE	HOME PHONE NO.

MOTHER'S EMPLOYER	OCCUPATION	HOW LONG EMPLOYED?	BUSINESS PHONE NO.

EMPLOYER'S STREET ADDRESS	CITY AND STATE	ZIP CODE

FATHER'S NAME	STREET ADDRESS, CITY, STATE AND ZIP CODE	HOME PHONE NO.

FATHER'S EMPLOYER	OCCUPATION	HOW LONG EMPLOYED?	BUSINESS PHONE NO.

EMPLOYER'S STREET ADDRESS	CITY AND STATE	ZIP CODE

INSURANCE INFORMATION

PERSON RESPONSIBLE FOR PAYMENT, IF NOT ABOVE	STREET ADDRESS, CITY, STATE AND ZIP CODE		HOME PHONE NO.
☐ COMPANY NAME & ADDRESS	NAME OF POLICYHOLDER	CERTIFICATE NO.	GROUP NO.
☐ COMPANY NAME & ADDRESS	NAME OF POLICYHOLDER	POLICY NO.	
☐ COMPANY NAME & ADDRESS	NAME OF POLICYHOLDER	POLICY NO.	

☐ MEDICARE	MEDICARE NO.	☐ MEDICAID	PROGRAM NO.	COUNTY NO.	ACCOUNT NO.

In order to control our cost of billing, we request that office visits be paid at the time service is rendered. We would rather control our billing costs than be forced to raise our fees.

AUTHORIZATION: I hereby authorize the physician indicated above to furnish information to insurance carriers concerning this illness/accident, and I hereby irrevocably assign to the doctor all payments for medical services rendered. I understand that I am financially responsible for all charges whether or not covered by insurance.

Responsible Party Signature

Equipment and Supplies

Statistical data sheet, pen or typewriter

NOTE: If a computer program is used to complete records, follow the instructions provided with the software. Basic principles provided in this procedure are still followed when information is entered into the computer.

Procedure

1. Assemble equipment. Use a private area for questioning the patient (lab partner in a practice situation).

   NOTE: A separate room with the door closed is preferred.

   CAUTION: Patient information is confidential. The patient's legal right to privacy must be observed.

2. Complete the statistical data sheet on page 44. Ask questions in a polite manner. Speak clearly and distinctly.

3. Type or print the name clearly. Check spelling.

4. Fill in the complete address of the patient's permanent residence. Use the space provided.

5. List the full telephone number of the patient's residence. If the patient does not have a telephone, put "none." Do not leave blank because doing so indicates that you have omitted the question. If the phone number is not local, list the area code.

6. Fill in the personal information requested, including age, full birthdate (month, day, and year), and sex.

7. Circle either *S*, *M*, *W*, or *D* to indicate the patient's marital status. The letters stand for *single*, *married*, *widowed*, or *divorced*.

8. List the patient's full Social Security number, placing dashes (-) between sections of the number (for example, 218-40-2593).

   CAUTION: Repeat and check numbers for accuracy.

9. List the spouse's name (the name of the patient's husband or wife), if this is requested. If the patient is single, widowed, or divorced, put "NA" for "not applicable."

10. List the patient's place of employment. Include address, telephone number, and other information requested. If the patient is not employed, put "none" or current work status such as "student" or "homemaker."

11. List the full name of the person responsible for the account. If this is the patient, list "self." If it is a husband, wife, or parent, complete all requested information.

12. List the full name of the insurance company and the company's address and telephone number. Double-check the policy number to be sure it is accurate. This information is essential for billing.

    NOTE: Be sure to include dashes, letters, and other parts of the policy number.

    NOTE: Most agencies make a copy of both the front and back of the patient's insurance card to place in the patient's file.

13. In the *referred by* section, place the name of the person who suggested your agency to the patient. This could be another physician, another patient, a friend, a relative, or even the telephone directory.

14. Recheck the information on the statistical data sheet as needed. Be sure all information is printed, typed, or keyed into a computer correctly. If an error occurs on a printed paper copy, draw a single red line through any incorrect entry and put your initials and the date near the line. Then insert the correct information. If an incorrect entry is noted on a computer page, delete the information and replace it with correct information.

Procedure 4:5 (cont.)

15. Replace all equipment.

Practice *Use the evaluation sheet for 4:5, Completing a Statistical Data Sheet, to practice this procedure. When you feel you have mastered this skill, sign the sheet and give it to your instructor for further action.*

✔ **Final Checkpoint** Using the criteria listed on the evaluation sheet, your instructor will grade your performance.

4:5 EVALUATION SHEET

Name _____ Date _____

Evaluated by _____

DIRECTIONS: Practice completing a statistical data sheet according to the criteria listed. When you are ready for your final check, give this sheet to your instructor.

Completing a Statistical Data Sheet	Points Possible	Yes	No	Points Earned	Comments
1. Assembles equipment	5				
2. Questions patient in a private area	8				
3. Asks questions politely	8				
4. Speaks clearly and distinctly	8				
5. Rechecks and repeats numbers for accuracy	8				
6. Types, keys, or prints all information neatly and legibly	8				
7. Completes all parts of the sheet with accurate information	10				
8. Uses correct abbreviations	8				
9. Avoids blanks—uses "none or "NA"	8				
10. Draws red line through error, initials, and inserts correct information	8				
11. Rechecks form at end to be sure all information is complete and accurate	8				
12. Notes any additional pertinent information the patient relates	8				
13. Replaces all equipment	5				
Totals	100				

4:6 ADMITTING A PATIENT

OBRA As a health care worker in a hospital or long-term care facility, one of your responsibilities may be to admit patients or residents. Although this procedure varies slightly in different facilities, basic principles apply in all facilities.

Admission to a health care facility can cause anxiety and fear in many patients and their families. The individual has to adjust to a new environment. It is important for the health care worker to create a positive first impression. By being courteous, supportive, and kind, the health care worker can do much to relieve fear and anxiety. Giving clear instructions on how to operate equipment and on the type of routine to expect helps the patient or resident become familiar with the environment. It is also important not to rush while admitting a patient. Allow the individual to ask questions and to express concerns. If you do not know the answers to specific questions, refer these questions to your immediate supervisor.

Most facilities have a specific form that is used during an admission. The form lists the procedures that must be performed and will vary slightly from facility to facility. It is important for the health care worker to become familiar with the information required on such forms. Much of the information on an admission form is used as a basis for the nursing care plan. Therefore, this information must be complete and accurate.

An admission form is a medical record. All information is confidential. No information can be released from this record without the written consent of the patient. In addition, since the admission form is a legal record, information must be printed or typed in a legible form. Spelling and punctuation must be correct. If an error is made while completing the admission form, the error should be crossed out in red ink, dated, and initialed. Correct information is then recorded.

The patient (or person providing the information) must have privacy while being questioned. A separate room should be used, and the door to the room should be closed. It is important that questions are asked in a professional manner. The patient must understand the meaning of all questions and should be given time to think about each question.

If the patient is unable to answer the questions, a relative or the person responsible for the patient is usually able to provide the information. An interpreter may be needed if a patient has limited English and speaks a foreign language.

In some facilities, questions regarding medications and allergies are the responsibility of the nurse. Follow agency policy regarding these sections on the form.

When a patient is admitted to a facility, certain procedures are performed. These usually include taking vital signs, measuring height and weight, and collecting a routine urine specimen. Follow correct techniques while performing these procedures.

In order to protect a patient's possessions, a personal inventory list is made of clothing, valuables, and personal items. In a hospital, a family member frequently will take clothing home. Any clothing or personal items (such as radios) kept in the room should be noted on the list. The list should be checked and signed by both the health care worker and the patient (or the person responsible for the patient). At the time of discharge, the personal inventory list of clothing and personal items should be checked to make sure that the patient has all belongings.

If the family does not take valuables home, these should be put in a safe place. Most facilities require that they be kept in a safe. A description of the valuables is usually written on a valuables envelope, and the items are placed inside. If money is left in the patient's wallet, it should be counted and the exact amount recorded on the envelope. Both the health care worker and the patient (or the person responsible for the patient) should check the items and sign the valuables envelope. The valuables are then put in the safe. A receipt is given to the patient or put on the patient's chart. If a patient is discharged, the valuables are taken from the safe and checked by both the health care worker and the patient. Again, both individuals sign the envelope to indicate that valuables have been returned to the patient.

Patients and family members should be oriented to the facility. Things they should be told include:

■ How to operate the call signal, bed controls, television remote control (if present), telephone, and other similar equipment

■ Visiting hours

■ Location of lounges

■ Smoking regulations

■ Availability of services such as religious services and activities

■ Mealtimes, and other rules or routines in the facility

Many facilities give patients and family members pamphlets or papers listing such information, but it is still important to explain the main information.

STUDENT: *Complete the assignment sheet for 4:6, Admitting a Patient. Then continue with the procedure.*

4:6 ADMITTING A PATIENT

ASSIGNMENT SHEET

Grade _____ Name _____

INTRODUCTION: This assignment will help you review the main facts about admitting a patient.

INSTRUCTIONS: Read the information on Admitting a Patient. In the space provided, print the word(s) that best completes the statement or answers the question.

1. Admission to a health care facility can cause _____ and _____ for many patients/residents and their families.

2. Identify two (2) ways a health care assistant can create a positive first impression and alleviate a patient's fears and anxiety.

3. If you make an error while completing an admission form, what should you do?

4. What must be obtained before any information is released from an admission form?

5. If a patient is unable to answer questions for an admission form, who can you ask for the information?

6. What should you do if a patient has limited English and speaks a foreign language?

7. List at least three (3) rules to follow while handling a patient's valuables.

8. List at least five (5) areas or things that should be explained while orientating a patient to the health care facility.

9. Interview a "patient" (your lab partner or another adult) who is entering the hospital for knee surgery. Complete the following admission form.

Name _____

ADMISSION FORM

PATIENT PREFERS TO BE ADDRESSED AS:

_____

FROM: ❑ E.R. ❑ E.C.F. ❑ Home ❑ M.D.'s Office

COMMUNICATES IN ENGLISH: ❑ Well ❑ Minimal ❑ Not At All ❑ Other Language (Specify) _____

❑ INTERPRETER (Name Person) ❑ None

_____

MODE OF TRANSPORTATION:

❑ Ambulatory ❑ Other Smoker: Y❑ N❑
❑ Wheelchair _____
❑ Stretcher _____

Home Telephone No. ( ) _____

Work Telephone No. ( ) _____

ORIENTATION TO ENVIRONMENT:

❑ Armband Checked ❑ Call Light
❑ Bed Control ❑ Phone
❑ TV Control ❑ Side Rail Policy
❑ Bath Room ❑ Visitation Policy
❑ Personal Property Policy ❑ Smoking Policy

PERSONAL BELONGINGS: (Check and Describe)

❑ Clothing _____
❑ Jewelry _____
❑ Money _____
❑ Walker _____
❑ Wheelchair _____
❑ Cane _____
❑ Other _____

DENTURES:

❑ Upper ❑ Partial
❑ Lower ❑ None

CONTACT LENSES:

❑ Hard ❑ LT ❑ RT
❑ Soft

GLASSES: ❑ Y ❑ N   **HEARING AID:** ❑ Y ❑ N

PROSTHESIS: ❑ Y ❑ N

(Describe) _____

DISPOSITION OF VALUABLES:

❑ Patient   Given To: _____
❑ Home
❑ Placed in   Relationship: _____
Safe
(Claim No.) _____

IN CASE OF EMERGENCY NOTIFY:

Name: _____

Relationship: _____

Home Telephone No. ( ) _____

Work Telephone No. ( ) _____

VITAL SIGNS:

TEMP: _____ ❑ Oral ❑ Rectal ❑ Axillary

PULSE: _____ ❑ Radial ❑ Apical Respiratory
Rate _____

❑ RT
B/P: _____ ❑ LT ❑ Standing ❑ Sitting ❑ Lying

HEIGHT: _____ WEIGHT: _____ ❑ Bedside
❑ Standing

ALLERGIES:

Medications: ❑ None Known   Food: ❑ None Known
❑ Penicillin ❑ Tape
❑ Sulfa ❑ Other (List) (Shellfish, Eggs, Milk, etc.)
❑ Iodine _____ _____
❑ Aspirin _____ _____
❑ Morphine _____ _____
❑ Demerol _____ _____

MEDICATIONS: (Prescription Non-Prescription) Dose/Frequency Last Dose (Date/Time)

1. _____ _____ _____
2. _____ _____ _____
3. _____ _____ _____
4. _____ _____ _____
5. _____ _____ _____
6. _____ _____ _____

DISPOSITION OF MEDICATIONS:

❑ None Brought to Hospital
❑ Sent Home _____
With _____
❑ To Pharmacy: (List)
_____
_____

ADMITTING DIAGNOSIS: _____

NURSE'S SIGNATURE: _____ RN/LVN Date _____ Time _____

PROCEDURE 4:6 ADMITTING A PATIENT

Equipment and Supplies

Admission form and/or personal inventory list, valuables envelope, admission kit (if used), thermometer, stethoscope, sphygmomanometer, watch with second hand, scale, patient gown (if needed), paper, pen or pencil

Procedure

1. Obtain orders from your immediate supervisor or check orders to obtain permission for the procedure.

2. Wash hands.

3. Assemble equipment. Prepare the room for the admission. Fanfold the top bed linen down to open the bed. If an admission kit is used, unpack the kit and place the items in the bedside stand or table. The admission kit usually includes a water pitcher, cup, soap dish, bar of soap, lotion, and mouthwash. Check the room to be sure all equipment and supplies are in their proper places.

4. You may be required to go to the admissions office to get the new patient or resident, or the patient may be brought to the room by other personnel.

5. Greet and identify the patient. Ask the patient if he or she prefers to be called by a particular name. Introduce yourself to the patient and to any family members present.
   NOTE: Be friendly and courteous at all times. Do not rush or hurry the patient.

6. Ask the family or visitors to wait in the lounge or lobby while you complete the admission process, if this is facility policy.
   NOTE: If a patient is not able to answer questions, a family member or other person responsible for the patient can remain in the room to complete the admission process.

7. Close the door and screen the unit. Ask the patient to change into a gown or pajamas. Assist the patient as necessary.
   NOTE: In long-term care facilities, residents usually wear street clothes during the day. In this case, gowns or pajamas are not used.

8. Position the patient comfortably in the bed or in a chair.

9. Complete the admission form on page 51. Ask questions slowly and clearly. Provide time for the patient to answer the questions.
   NOTE: Observe the patient carefully during the admission process. Record all observations noted. If the patient expresses certain concerns, be sure to record and report these concerns.

10. Measure and record vital signs. Follow the procedures outlined in Chapter 12.

11. Weigh and measure the patient. Record the information on the admission form.

12. Complete a personal inventory list. Be sure to list all personal items that will be kept in the patient's unit such as clothing, shoes, clocks, radios, religious items, and books. Make sure the patient or a responsible individual checks and signs the list. Assist the patient as necessary in hanging up clothing or putting away personal items.

13. Complete a valuables list. If a family member takes the valuables home, be sure to obtain a signature on the proper form. If the valuables are to be placed in a safe, fill out the form and obtain the patient's and/or a relative's signature. Follow agency policy for placing the valuables in the safe.

14. Orient the patient to the facility by demonstrating or explaining the following:
    a. Call signal or light
    b. Bed controls
    c. Television remote control and/or television rental policy
    d. Telephone

Procedure 4:6 (cont.)

    e. Bathroom facilities and special call signal in bathroom

    f. Visiting hours

    g. Mealtimes and menu selections

    h. Activities or services available

15. Fill the water pitcher, if the patient is allowed to have liquids.

16. Observe all checkpoints before leaving the patient. Make sure the patient is comfortable and in good body alignment; the siderails are up, if indicated; the bed is at its lowest level; the call signal and supplies are in easy reach; and the area is neat and clean.

17. Clean and replace all equipment.

18. Wash hands.

19. When the admission process is complete, allow family members to return to the unit. Answer any questions they may have regarding facility policies. If you do not know answers to their questions, obtain the correct answers from your immediate supervisor.

20. Record all required information on the patient's chart or the agency form, for example, date; time; admission form complete, valuables placed in safe, patient tolerated procedure well; and your signature and title. Report any abnormal observations to your immediate supervisor.

Practice *Use the evaluation sheet for 4:6, Admitting a Patient, to practice this procedure. When you feel you have mastered this skill, sign the sheet and give it to your instructor for further action.*

✔ **Final Checkpoint** Using the criteria listed on the evaluation sheet, your instructor will grade your performance.

Name _____ Date _____

Evaluated by _____

DIRECTIONS: Practice admitting a patient according to the criteria listed. When you are ready for your final check, give this sheet to your instructor.

Admitting a Patient	Points Possible	Yes	No	Points Earned	Comments
1. Checks orders or obtains authorization	3				
2. Washes hands	3				
3. Assembles equipment and supplies	3				
4. Prepares room for admission:					
Opens the bed	3				
Unpacks admission kit	3				
Places supplies/equipment in bedside stand	3				
5. Greets and identifies patient	4				
6. Introduces self	4				
7. Asks family/visitors to wait in lounge/lobby	4				
8. Closes door and screens unit	4				
9. Assists patient into gown/pajamas	4				
10. Positions patient comfortably in bed/chair	4				
11. Completes admission form/checklist	4				
12. Measures and records vital signs	4				
13. Weighs and measures patient	4				
14. Completes personal inventory list:					
Lists personal items	3				
Obtains proper signatures	3				
Hangs up clothes and puts items away	3				
15. Completes valuables list:					
Obtains proper signatures	3				
Places valuables in safe	3				
16. Orientates patient to facility	4				
17. Fills water pitcher if allowed	4				
18. Positions patient in correct alignment	4				
19. Elevates siderail if indicated and lowers bed before leaving patient	3				

Evaluation 4:6 (cont.)

Admitting a Patient	Points Possible	Yes	No	Points Earned	Comments
20. Places call signal and supplies in patient's reach	3				
21. Replaces equipment and leaves area neat and clean	3				
22. Washes hands	3				
23. Allows family/visitors to return to unit	3				
24. Records or reports required information	4				
Totals	100				

OBRA Height and weight measurements are taken in many health care fields. Height and weight measurements are used to determine whether a patient is overweight or underweight. Either of these conditions can indicate disease. Height–weight charts are used as averages. A 10 percent deviation is usually considered normal. Height–weight measurements must be accurate. Always recheck your calculations.

Height–weight measurements are usually routinely done when a patient is admitted to a hospital, long-term care facility, or other health care agency. They are also a part of the general physical examination in a physician's office. In addition, the measurements provide necessary information in performing and evaluating certain laboratory tests and in calculating dosages of certain medications.

The height, weight, and head circumference measurements of infants and toddlers are monitored frequently because growth is rapid. Usually infants are checked every two months to detect any changes that may indicate problems with growth and development. The measurements are usually recorded on a National Center for Health Statistics (NCHS) growth graph (see page 57). The graphed information allows the physician to check the child's growth and compare it with the average percentiles of other children the same age. Abnormal growth patterns may indicate nutritional deficiencies or genetic diseases.

Patients with cancer or patients on chemotherapy are weighed frequently to monitor weight loss. Daily weights are often ordered for patients with edema (swelling) due to heart, kidney, or other diseases. When taking daily weights, note the following points:

- Use the same scale each day.

- Make sure the scale is balanced before weighing the patient.

- Weigh the patient at the same time each day.

- Make sure the patient is wearing the same amount of clothing each day.

! Careful consideration must be given to the safety of the patient while weight and height are being measured. Observe the patient closely at all times. Prevent falls from the scale and possible injury from the protruding height lever.

C Most patients are very weight conscious. Parents may worry about the weight of their children. Therefore, it is very important for the health care worker to make only positive statements while weighing a patient. In addition, privacy must be provided while weighing a patient.

A wide variety of scales are used to obtain height and weight measurements. Most clinical scales contain a balance beam for measuring weight and a measuring rod for determining height. Infant scales provide an area for placing the infant in a lying-down, or flat, position.

≋ Weight is recorded as pounds and ounces or as kilograms (1.0 kilogram = 2.2 pounds). Most scales measure pounds in ¼-pound increments. Metric scales measure in kilograms and have 0.1-kilogram increments.

Height is recorded as feet and inches or as centimeters. The measuring bar measures inches and fractions or ¼-inch increments. A metric measuring bar has 1-centimeter increments. One inch equals 2.5 centimeters.

STUDENT: *Complete the assignment sheet for 4:7, Measuring/Recording Height and Weight. Then continue with the procedure.*

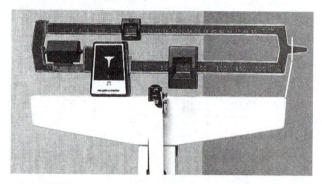

The weight bars. The bottom weights are in 50-pound increments, and the top weights are in ¼-pound increments.

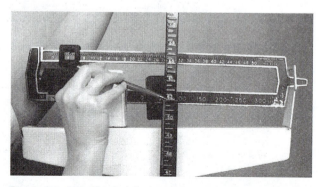

The height bar. The height is read at the break-point on the movable bar.

Birth to 36 months: Boys
Length-for-age and Weight-for-age percentiles

NAME ____________________

RECORD # ____________

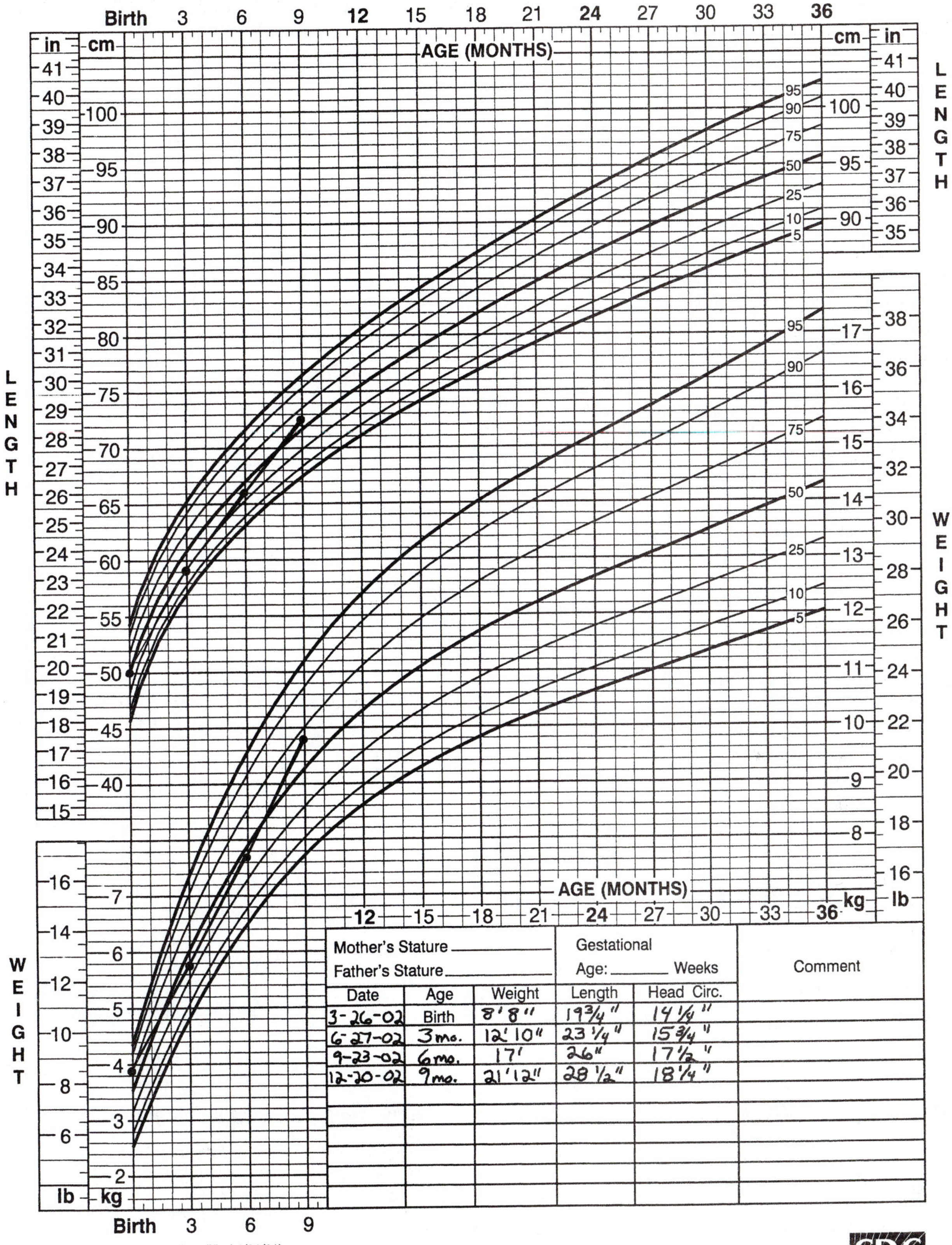

Mother's Stature			Gestational Age: ____ Weeks		Comment
Father's Stature					
Date	Age	Weight	Length	Head Circ.	
3-26-02	Birth	8'8"	19¾"	14¼"	
6-27-02	3mo.	12'10"	23¼"	15¾"	
9-23-02	6mo.	17'	26"	17½"	
12-20-02	9mo.	21'12"	28½"	18¼"	

Published May 30, 2000 (modified 4/20/01).
SOURCE: Developed by the National Center for Health Statistics in collaboration with the National Center for Chronic Disease Prevention and Health Promotion (2000).
http://www.cdc.gov/growthcharts

CDC
SAFER • HEALTHIER • PEOPLE™

The National Center for Health Statistics (NCHS) growth graph is used to monitor the growth and development of infants and toddlers.

ASSIGNMENT SHEET

Grade _____ Name _____

INTRODUCTION: This assignment will help you review the main facts regarding measuring/recording height and weight.

INSTRUCTIONS: Review the information on Measuring/Recording Height and Weight. In the space provided, print the word(s) that best completes the statement or answers the question.

1. Height and weight measurements are used to determine whether a patient is _____ or _____. A _____ deviation is usually considered normal.

2. Identify two (2) times height-weight measurements may be done.

3. Why are an infant's height, weight, and head circumference measurements checked every two months?

4. List two (2) points that must be followed if daily weights are done on a patient.

5. Why should the patient be observed closely at all times while weight and height are being measured?

6. Why is it important to make only positive statements while weighing a patient?

7. The large weight on a scale is set at 50 pounds. The small weight is set at 23 pounds. How much does the patient weigh?

8. The large weight on a scale is set at 150 pounds. The small weight is set at 41½ pounds. How much does the patient weigh?

9. The height bar shows a height of 62 inches. How tall is the patient in feet and inches? (*Hint:* Divide by 12 because there are 12 inches in one foot.)

10. The height bar shows a height of 49½ inches. How tall is the patient in feet and inches?

PROCEDURE 4:7 MEASURING/RECORDING HEIGHT AND WEIGHT

Equipment and Supplies

Balance scale, paper towel, paper, pencil or pen

Procedure

1. Assemble equipment.

2. Wash hands.

3. Prepare the scale. Place a paper towel on the foot stand of the scale. Move both weights to the *zero* position. If the end of the balance bar swings freely, the scale is balanced. If the scale is *not* balanced, follow manufacturer's instructions to balance the scale.

   NOTE: Most scales have a small screw by the end of the balance bar. By adjusting the screw, the scale can be balanced.

   NOTE: The paper towel prevents spread of disease.

4. Introduce yourself. Identify the patient. Explain the procedure. Remember to make only positive statements.

5. Ask the patient to remove shoes, jackets, heavy outer clothing, purses, and heavy objects that may be in the pockets of clothing.

   NOTE: In a hospital or long-term care facility, the patient is usually weighed in a gown or in pajamas.

6. Assist the patient onto the scale. The patient should stand unassisted, with his or her feet centered on the platform and slightly apart.

   CAUTION: Watch closely at all times to prevent falls.

7. Move the large 50-pound weight to the right until the balance bar drops down on the lower guide. Then move this weight back one notch. Move the smaller ¼-pound weight until the balance bar swings freely halfway between the upper and lower guides. Add the two weights together to determine the patient's correct weight. Recheck your reading. Record the weight correctly.

8. Help the patient get off the scale. Raise the height bar higher than the height of the patient. Help the patient get back on the scale with his or her back to the scale.

   CAUTION: Watch closely at all times to prevent falls.

9. Instruct the patient to stand as erect as possible.

10. Move the bar of the measuring scale down until it just touches the top of the patient's head.

    CAUTION: Move slowly. Do *not* hit the patient with the bar.

11. Read the measurement in inches or centimeters. Recheck your reading. Record the height correctly.

    NOTE: If the height is difficult to read, assist the patient off the scale without moving the height bar. Then read the correct height measurement.

    NOTE: If the reading is in inches, it can be converted to feet and inches after the patient is off the scale.

    NOTE: If the height bar is extended above the break point of the movable bar, remember to read the height at the point of the break by reading in a downward direction on the upper bar.

12. Elevate the height bar.

13. Help the patient get off the scale.

    CAUTION: Watch the patient closely to prevent falls.

14. Replace all equipment. Throw the paper towel in a waste can.

Procedure 4:7 (cont.)

15. Return both weight beams to the zero positions. Lower the measurement bar.

16. Convert the inches to feet and inches by dividing by 12. For example 64½ inches divided by 12 equals 5 feet 4½ inches.

17. Wash hands.

18. Record all required information on the patient's chart, for example, date, time, Wt: 132½ lb, Ht: 5 ft 4½ in., and your signature and title.

Practice *Use the evaluation sheet for 4:7, Measuring/Recording Height and Weight, to practice this procedure. When you feel you have mastered this skill, sign the sheet and give it to your instructor for further action.*

✔ **Final Checkpoint** Using the criteria listed on the evaluation sheet, your instructor will grade your performance.

4:7 EVALUATION SHEET

Name _____ Date _____

Evaluated by _____

DIRECTIONS: Practice measuring height and weight according to the criteria listed. When you are ready for your final check, give this sheet to your instructor.

Measuring/Recording Height and Weight	Points Possible	Yes	No	Points Earned	Comments
1. Assembles equipment and supplies	3				
2. Washes hands	3				
3. Places paper towel on foot platform of scale	3				
4. Balances scale at zero	3				
5. Introduces self, identifies patient, and explains procedure	3				
6. Tells patient to remove shoes, jackets, heavy outer clothing, purses, and heavy objects in pocket	3				
7. Positions patient on scale:					
Assists as needed	2				
Positions in center of platform	2				
Positions feet slightly apart	2				
Checks that patient is standing unassisted	2				
8. Balances scale correctly	4				
9. Reads weight correctly	6				
10. Records weight correctly	6				
11. Assists patient off of scale	4				
12. Raises height bar	4				
13. Assists patient back onto scale with back toward scale	4				
14. Asks patient to stand as erect as possible	4				
15. Moves measuring bar without hitting patient	4				
16. Positions bar correctly	4				
17. Accurately reads measurement in inches	6				
18. Assists patient off scale after elevating height bar	4				
19. Converts height measurement to feet and inches	6				
20. Records height correctly	6				
21. Replaces all equipment	3				
22. Returns weight beams to zero	3				
23. Lowers measurement bar	3				
24. Washes hands	3				
Totals	100				

4:8 PART 1: MENTAL HEALTH MYTHS TEST

People's reactions to mental and emotional disorders are often different from their reactions to physical illnesses. Part of this difference is due to many myths, or false beliefs, about mental illness. These myths have existed throughout history. Years ago, people who were "different" were frequently locked behind bars in mental institutions. Treatment was limited to confinement and separation from others. Today, treatment for mental and emotional disorders is much improved. Medications can control many conditions. Counseling can help individuals lead productive lives. However, even though major advances have been made in treating mental and emotional disorders, many myths still exist.

Do you believe some of these myths? Take the test on *Your Knowledge of Mental Illness*. After you complete the test, use the answer key to grade your knowledge. Do you need to make an effort to learn more about mental illness?

4:8 YOUR KNOWLEDGE OF MENTAL ILLNESS TEST

ASSIGNMENT SHEET

Grade _____ Name _____

INSTRUCTIONS: In the space provided by each question, write "true" if you feel the statement is true and "false" if you feel the statement is false.

_____ 1. Only crazy people have a mental illness.

_____ 2. Mental illness is something that happens only to adults.

_____ 3. Everyone with a mental illness must be treated in a mental hospital.

_____ 4. People with mental illness are not in touch with reality.

_____ 5. You can treat mental illness yourself if you just work through the problem.

_____ 6. People with mental health problems are usually violent.

_____ 7. You can prevent someone from committing suicide by telling the person you don't care if he or she does it.

_____ 8. A person who says "I'm going to kill myself" will not do it.

_____ 9. A person with depression must take medicine his or her entire life to keep from getting depressed.

_____ 10. Mental illness only gets worse as a person ages.

Answers to Your Knowledge of Mental Illness Test

1. False: Mental illness, like many others forms of illness, can range from mild to severe. The term "crazy" has no place in reference to mental illness.

2. False: Mental illness, like most other illnesses, can occur at any age.

3. False: Most people with mental illness are treated without ever being admitted to a hospital.

4. False: People with mental illness are in touch with reality. A few people with severe and untreated mental illness may lose touch with reality.

5. False: Psychological problems almost always require the help of a health care professional.

6. False: People with mental illness are usually not violent. Some may exhibit violence as a result of their illness, but most behaviors can be controlled with treatment.

7. False: Never challenge a person to commit suicide. The person needs you to listen and offer support so you can help him or her obtain help with the problem.

8. False: A person who states he or she will kill himself or herself is crying for help. It is important to make sure the person finds someone who can help with the problems.

9. False: Many cases of depression are relieved by medication and counseling. After treatment the individual does not need medication.

10. False: Mental illness can improve with age as a person matures and learns to handle problems. In some cases, without treatment or help, it can become worse.

Summary: All 10 questions are common myths about mental illness. Did you believe these myths? How did you rate on your knowledge of mental illness?

9 to 10 Correct Answers: You are well informed and have a healthy attitude about mental illness.

7 to 8 Correct Answers: You have a good basic knowledge about mental illness but need to learn more.

6 Correct Answers: Your knowledge about mental illness is fair. You still believe some common myths. Try to learn the truth about mental illness.

Below 5: You believe too many myths on mental illness. Study hard to learn the truth.

4:8 PART 2: HOW DO OTHERS SEE YOU?

Mental and social services workers perform many types of assessments to find out about an individual. The assessments can range from simple personality tests to complex psychological evaluations. The purpose of the assessments is to determine how an individual reacts or responds. This knowledge can be beneficial during counseling or treatment. Many assessment tests do not have right or wrong answers. The tests just indicate what an individual likes or dislikes. The test results allow a professional to provide individualized treatment.

A simple assessment titled *How Do Others See You?* is provided. This is a sample of a test that has no *right* or *wrong* answers. It simply gives you a general idea of how others may see you. It is important to note that your own responses to this assessment may vary from time to time. If you take the test while you are feeling happy and confident, your answers may be slightly different than if you take the test while you are sad or discouraged. Remember, this is just one simple way to obtain information about your individual likes or dislikes.

Take the assessment. Then use the answer key that has been provided to obtain your score. Check the meaning of the scores. Do they seem to describe you? Why or why not?

4:8 How Do Others See You? Assessment

ASSIGNMENT SHEET

Grade _____ Name _____

INSTRUCTIONS: Circle the letter of the answer that best answers the question or describes your responses.

1. When do you feel your best?
   a. in the morning
   b. during the afternoon or early evening
   c. late at night

2. You usually walk
   a. fairly fast with long steps
   b. fairly fast with little steps
   c. at a medium pace with your head up
   d. slowly with your head down
   e. very slowly

3. When you talk to people you
   a. stand with your arms folded or relaxed at your side
   b. have your hands clasped together
   c. have one or both of your hands on your hips
   d. touch or stand very close to the person to whom you are talking
   e. play with your ear, touch your chin, or smooth your hair

4. When you relax, you sit with
   a. your knees bent with your legs side by side
   b. your legs crossed
   c. your legs stretched straight in front of you
   d. one leg curled under you

5. When something really amuses you, you react with
   a. a big hardy loud laugh
   b. a hardy laugh, but not a loud one
   c. a quiet chuckle
   d. a medium loud laugh
   e. a sheepish smile

6. When you arrive at a party or social gathering, you
   a. make a loud entrance so everyone notices you
   b. make a quiet entrance and look around for your friends or someone you know
   c. make a quiet entrance and try to stay unnoticed

7. You are working very hard and concentrating on your work. Someone interrupts. You
   a. welcome the break
   b. feel extremely irritated or mad
   c. vary between the two extremes

8. Which of the following colors do you like the most?
   a. red or orange
   b. black
   c. yellow or light blue
   d. green
   e. dark blue or purple
   f. white
   g. brown or gray

9. When you are in bed at night, the position you use to sleep is
   a. stretched out flat on your back
   b. stretched out face down on your stomach
   c. on your side, slightly curled
   d. on your side with your head on one arm
   e. with your head under the covers

10. You often dream that you are
    a. falling
    b. fighting or struggling
    c. searching for something or somebody
    d. flying or floating
    e. you usually do not dream
    f. your dreams are always pleasant

Assessment Answers

INSTRUCTIONS: Use the key below to obtain your score.

1. a. 2   b. 4   c. 6
2. a. 6   b. 4   c. 7   d. 2   e. 1
3. a. 4   b. 2   c. 5   d. 7   e. 6
4. a. 4   b. 6   c. 2   d. 1
5. a. 6   b. 4   c. 3   d. 5   e. 2
6. a. 6   b. 4   c. 2
7. a. 6   b. 2   c. 4
8. a. 6   b. 7   c. 5   d. 4   e. 3   f. 2   g. 1
9. a. 7   b. 6   c. 4   d. 2   e. 1
10. a. 4   b. 2   c. 3   d. 5   e. 6   f. 1

Summary: Add the total number of points to obtain your score. Now compare your score with the descriptions below:

Over 60 Points: Others see you as someone they should "handle with care." They may think you are vain, self-centered, and extremely dominant. Others may admire you and wish they could be more like you. However, they may not always trust you.

51 to 60 Points: Others see you as an exciting, rather impulsive personality. They think you are a natural leader, a person who is quick to make decisions, even though the decisions may not always be the right ones. They see you as bold, willing to try anything once, ready to take chances, and adventuresome. They enjoy your company because of the excitement you create.

41 to 50 Points: Others see you as fresh, lively, charming, amusing, practical, and interesting. They feel you are a person who is the center of attention but well balanced and not conceited. They feel you are kind, considerate, and understanding. They know you will always cheer them up or help them out.

31 to 40 Points: Others see you as sensible, cautious, careful, and practical. They think you are clever, gifted, and talented, but modest. They may feel you are a person who does not make friends quickly or easily, but they know that you are extremely loyal to friends you do make and that you expect the same loyalty in return. If they really get to know you, they realize it takes a lot for you to lose your trust in a friend but that if you do lose the trust, it will take you a long time to get over it.

21 to 30 Points: Your friends see you as painstaking and fussy. They feel you are very cautious and extremely careful but slow and steady. They would be surprised if you ever did something impulsively or on the spur of the moment. They expect you to examine everything carefully and make a well-informed decision. They know that if you decide to support or help them, you will follow through.

Under 21 Points: Others feel you are shy, nervous, and indecisive. They feel you are someone who needs looking after, someone who needs others to make decisions, and someone who does not like to get involved. They see you as a worrier who always sees problems that don't exist. A few people may think you are boring. Those who know you well know that you can be a good friend and provide support and understanding.

4:9 WRITING AN OBITUARY

One major job performed by an individual working in a mortuary career is to write an obituary. An obituary is a notice of a person's death. Most obituaries are found in newspapers. The most common type includes information such as:

- The individual's full name
- Date of birth and date of death
- Age at time of death
- Names of survivors including spouse (husband or wife), children, parents, sisters, and/or brothers
- Place of employment or, in the case of a young child, school(s) attended
- Military experience
- Organizations or associations the individual was involved with
- Time and place of funeral services
- How to make memorial contributions

Even though the above points provide the major facts about an individual, they do not reveal the special aspects of the person's life. As we go through life, each of us would like to be remembered for the things we believe in and the special things we do. These are the things that make us an individual. In order to learn about these unique aspects of a person's life, different questions must be asked. Examples of some other questions might include:

- What did the individual like to do?
- Was he or she involved in sports?
- Did he or she have any hobbies?
- Did the individual like to read, garden, cook gourmet foods, do woodworking, restore old cars, boat, fish, ride a bike, take photographs, or have other hobbies?
- Did the person do volunteer work at an animal shelter, homeless shelter, children's hospital, church, or community center?
- For what special achievement would the person want to be remembered?
- Did the person have a special pet? What was the pet's name?

The assignment that follows will allow you to write an obituary. Think about the above questions and try to write a tribute to a person's life. It is easy to list the basic facts. It is a little harder to write something that really describes the uniqueness of the individual. How would you like to be remembered?

4:9 WRITING AN OBITUARY

ASSIGNMENT SHEET

Grade _____ Name _____

INSTRUCTIONS: Read the information on Writing an Obituary. Look at the following list of suggested individuals and choose one person. In the space provided, write a tribute to that person's life.

1. A close friend

2. A parent

3. A sister or brother

4. An aunt or uncle

5. An adult whom you respect or admire

6. An individual who made a major contribution to health care

7. Yourself

4:10 TRANSFERRING A PATIENT TO A WHEELCHAIR

As a health care worker, you may be responsible for transferring a patient to a wheelchair. If you perform this procedure correctly, you will provide the patient with optimum comfort and care. In addition, you will prevent injury to yourself and the patient.

It is important to remember that an incorrect technique can result in serious injury to the patient. Some patients cannot be moved or transferred without special assistance or mechanical devices such as a patient lift. If a patient has restrictions for moving or transferring, every individual who works with the patient must be aware of the restrictions. If you are not sure a patient can be moved or transferred safely, *always* ask your supervisor before attempting any procedure. Remember, you are *legally* responsible for the safety and well-being of the patient.

Correct body mechanics are required for any transfer to a wheelchair. Review and practice all of the rules of correct body mechanics as outlined in Chapter 10:1. If you are unable to move a patient by yourself, always get help.

A wheelchair is a device that is frequently used to transport patients who are weak or not able to walk. There are many types of wheelchairs. Most contain large wheels with rubber treads to provide traction. Locks are provided for the wheels to prevent movement of the chair. The locks must be in position when a patient is getting in or out of the chair. Wheelchairs also have armrests and footrests. The armrests on some wheelchairs can be moved to the side to allow a patient to slide into the seat of the chair. The footrests are usually folded back while the patient is getting into the chair. After the patient is seated in the chair, the footrests are dropped into position to provide support for the patient's feet. Before using any wheelchair, it is important to read the manufacturer's instructions. If the instructions are not available, have someone in authority show you how to operate the chair.

A transfer belt is usually placed on a patient before the patient is moved to a wheelchair. The transfer belt is a band of fabric that is positioned around the patient's waist. During transfers, the health care worker can grasp the transfer belt to provide additional support for the patient. The belt helps provide the patient with a sense of security and helps to stabilize the patient's center of gravity. Some important points to remember when using a transfer belt include:

- The transfer belt must be the correct size. It should fit securely around the waist for support but must not be too tight for comfort.

- After the belt has been applied to the patient, the health care worker should place his or her hands under the belt to make sure it is not too tight.

- Some transfer belts contain loops that are grasped when moving the patient. If loops are not present, an underhand grasp should be used to hold on to the belt. The underhand grasp is more secure than grasping the belt from the top, because the hands are less likely to slip off the belt.

- When assisting a patient to stand, the health care assistant should face the patient and grasp the belt on both sides.

- The transfer belt is applied over the patient's clothing. It should not be applied over bare skin because it can irritate the skin.

Before a patient is moved or transferred, the health care worker must obtain approval or orders from his or her immediate supervisor. Never move or transfer a patient without correct authorization.

During any move or transfer, it is important to watch the patient closely. Note changes in pulse rate, respirations, and color. Observe for signs of weakness, dizziness, increased perspiration, or discomfort. If you see any abnormal changes, return the patient to a safe and comfortable position and check with your immediate supervisor. The supervisor will determine whether the move or transfer should be attempted.

STUDENT: *Complete the assignment sheet for 4:10, Transferring a Patient to a Wheelchair. Then continue with the procedure.*

4:10 TRANSFERRING A PATIENT TO A WHEELCHAIR

ASSIGNMENT SHEET

Grade _____ Name _____

INTRODUCTION: This assignment will help you review the main facts regarding transferring a patient to a wheelchair.

INSTRUCTIONS: Review the information on Transferring a Patient to a Wheelchair. In the space provided, print the word(s) that best completes the statement or answers the question.

1. What should you do if you are not sure a patient can be transferred to a wheelchair?

2. What is the purpose of the rubber treads on the wheels of a wheelchair?

3. When should the wheels on a wheelchair be locked?

4. If manufacturer's instructions are not available and you do not know how to operate a wheelchair, what should you do?

5. A transfer belt helps provide the patient with a sense of _____ and helps to stabilize the patient's _____.

6. You have just applied a transfer belt to a patient's waist. How can you make sure that the belt is not too tight?

7. If loops are not present on a transfer belt, what type of grasp should be used? Why?

8. List four (4) things that a health care worker should watch while transferring a patient to a wheelchair.

PROCEDURE 4:10 TRANSFERRING A PATIENT TO A WHEELCHAIR

NOTE: Wheelchairs vary slightly. Read the manufacturer's instructions or ask your immediate supervisor to demonstrate correct operation of the footrests, wheel locks, and other parts.

Equipment and Supplies

Wheelchair or chair, bathrobe, transfer belt, one to two bath blankets, slippers, pen or pencil

Procedure

1. Obtain orders from your immediate supervisor or check physician's orders to obtain authorization.

2. Assemble equipment.

3. Knock on the door and pause before entering. Introduce yourself. Identify the patient. Explain the procedure to the patient.

4. Close the door and screen the unit to provide privacy for the patient.

5. Wash hands.

6. Position the wheelchair. It can be placed at the head of the bed facing the foot or at the foot of the bed facing the head. Positioning often depends on other equipment in the room.
   NOTE: Whenever possible, the chair should be positioned so that it is secure against a wall or solid furniture and will *not* slide backward.

7. Securely lock the wheels of the wheelchair. Raise the footrests so that they are out of the way.
   CAUTION: Double-check the locks on the wheelchair.

   NOTE: For additional comfort and warmth, a bath blanket can be folded lengthwise and placed in the wheelchair.

8. Lock the bed to prevent movement. Lower the bed to its lowest level.

9. Slowly elevate the head of the bed.

10. Lower the siderail on the side that the patient is to exit from the bed.

11. Put the robe on the patient. Fanfold the bed linen to the foot of the bed.
    NOTE: Avoid exposing the patient during this procedure.

12. Assist the patient to a sitting position on the side of the bed with his or her feet flat on the floor. Observe for any signs of distress. Note color, pulse rate, breathing, and other similar signs. Put socks and shoes or slippers with nonslip soles on the patient. Put a transfer belt on the patient.
    CAUTION: If the patient is weak or too heavy, get help.

    CAUTION: If distress is noted, return the patient to bed immediately.

    CAUTION: Use proper body mechanics.

13. Keep your back straight. Place one hand on each side of the belt using an underhand grasp. Face the patient and stand close to the patient. Position your feet to provide a broad base of support. If the patient has a weak leg, support the leg by positioning your knee against the patient's knee or by blocking the patient's foot with your foot.
    NOTE: If the use of a transfer belt is contraindicated, place your hands under the patient's arms and around to the back of the shoulders to provide support.

14. Arrange a signal with the patient, such as counting to three. Instruct the patient to push against the bed with his or her hands to rise to a standing position.

Procedure 4:10 (cont.)

15. At the given signal, assist the patient to a standing position. Lift up on the belt while the patient pushes up from the bed. Place your knees and feet firmly against the patient's knees and feet to provide support.

16. Keeping your hands in the same position, help the patient turn by using several pivot steps until the back of his or her legs are touching the seat of the chair.

17. Ask the patient to place his or her hands on the armrests and to bend at the knees as you gradually and slowly lower the patient to a sitting position in the chair.

     CAUTION: Bend at the hips and knees and keep your back straight.

18. Position the patient comfortably. Remove the transfer belt. Use a bath blanket to cover the patient's lap and legs. Lower the footrests on the wheelchair, taking care not to hit the patient's feet.

    NOTE: Observe for any signs of distress.

19. Remain with the patient until you are sure there are no problems. If you leave the patient seated in a wheelchair or chair, make sure that the call signal and other supplies are within easy reach. Leave the area neat and clean. Check on the patient at frequent intervals.

20. If you are transporting the patient in the wheelchair, observe the following rules:

    a. Walk on the right side of the hall or corridor.

    b. Slow down and look for other traffic at doorways and intersections.

    c. To enter an elevator, turn the chair around and back into the elevator.

    d. To go down a steep ramp, turn the chair around and back down the ramp.

    e. Use the weight of your body to push the chair. Stand close to the chair.

    f. Watch the patient closely for signs of distress while transporting.

21. To return the patient to bed, reverse the procedure, beginning by putting a transfer belt on the patient and raising the footrests (step 18).

    CAUTION: Be sure the wheels are locked before helping the patient out of the wheelchair. Lock the bed to prevent movement.

22. Position the patient in good body alignment after returning him or her to bed.

23. Observe all checkpoints before leaving the patient: elevate the siderails (if indicated), lower the bed to its lowest level, place the call signal and other supplies within easy reach of the patient.

24. Replace all equipment used. Wipe the wheelchair with a disinfectant and return it to its proper place. Leave the area neat and clean.

25. Wash hands.

26. Report that the patient was transferred to a wheelchair and/or record all required information on the patient's chart or the agency form, for example, date; time; transferred to chair, sat in chair for 30 minutes, tolerated well; and your signature and title. Note any unusual observations.

Practice *Use the evaluation sheet for 4:10, Transferring a Patient to a Wheelchair, to practice this procedure. When you feel you have mastered this skill, sign the sheet and give it to your instructor for further action.*

✔ **Final Checkpoint** Using the criteria listed on the evaluation sheet, your instructor will grade your performance.

4:10 EVALUATION SHEET

Name _____ Date _____

Evaluated by _____

DIRECTIONS: Practice transferring patient to a wheelchair according to the criteria listed. When you are ready for your final check, give this sheet to your instructor.

Transferring a Patient to a Wheelchair	Points Possible	Yes	No	Points Earned	Comments
1. Checks order or obtains authorization	3				
2. Assembles equipment and supplies	2				
3. Knocks on door and pauses before entering	2				
4. Introduces self, identifies patient, and explains procedure	2				
5. Closes door and screens unit	2				
6. Washes hands	3				
7. Prepares wheelchair:					
Positions correctly	2				
Locks wheels	2				
Elevates footrests	2				
8. Locks bed to prevent movement	2				
9. Lowers bed to lowest level	2				
10. Elevates head slowly	2				
11. Lowers siderail (if elevated) on side patient will exit bed	2				
12. Assists patient to put on robe	2				
13. Assists patient to sitting position	3				
14. Puts transfer belt on patient	3				
15. Helps with slippers or shoes	2				
16. Stands close to patient with broad base of support	3				
17. Grasps each side of belt with underhand grasp	3				
18. Gives signal	3				
19. Assists to standing position by lifting up on belt while patient pushes up from the bed	4				
20. Allows patient to adjust to upright position	4				

Transferring a Patient to a Wheelchair	Points Possible	Yes	No	Points Earned	Comments
21. Turns patient to chair slowly and provides support for patient's leg(s) as needed	4				
22. Lowers gently into chair when patient's legs touch seat of chair	4				
23. Covers with blanket	3				
24. Observes for signs of distress	3				
25. Transports patient in wheelchair correctly:					
Direct wheelchair to right of hallway	3				
Watches intersections	3				
Pulls backward into elevator	3				
Walks backward down ramp	3				
Uses weight of body to push chair	3				
26. Returns patient to bed correctly	3				
27. Positions patient in correct alignment	2				
28. Elevates siderails if indicated and lowers bed to lowest level	2				
29. Places call signal and other supplies within reach of patient	2				
30. Replaces all equipment and leaves area neat and clean	2				
31. Washes hands	2				
32. Records or reports required information	3				
Totals	100				

4:11 FEEDING A PATIENT

OBRA Good nutrition is an important part of a patient's treatment. It may be one of your responsibilities to make mealtimes as pleasant as possible for the patient. Mealtimes are often regarded as a time for social interaction. Most people prefer to eat with others. People who eat alone often have poor appetites and poor nutrition. In long-term care facilities, patients are encouraged to eat in the dining room. This provides an opportunity for social interaction with others. If a patient is confined to bed, it is important to talk with the patient while serving the food tray or feeding the patient.

Proper mealtime preparation is important. If the patient is ready to eat when the tray arrives, mealtime is likely to be more pleasant. Preparation before the tray is delivered includes:

- Offering the bedpan or urinal or assisting the patient to the bathroom. Clear the room of any offensive odors by using a deodorizer or opening a window.

- Allowing the patient to wash his or her hands and face, if desired.

- Providing oral hygiene, if desired. Many individuals want to brush their teeth before meals, especially before breakfast.

- Positioning the patient comfortably and in a sitting position, if possible.

- Clearing the overbed table and positioning it for the tray.

- Removing objects such as an emesis basin or bedpan from the patient's view. Place such objects in the bedside stand, if they will not be needed.

If a meal will be delayed because of X-rays or other treatments, be sure to explain this to the patient.

Check the tray carefully against the patient's name and room number and the type of diet ordered. If anything seems out of place (for example, a salt shaker provided with a salt-free diet or sugar with a diabetic diet), check with your immediate supervisor or the dietitian. Never add any food to the tray without checking the diet order first.

Allow patients to feed themselves whenever possible. If necessary, assist by cutting meat, opening beverage cartons, and buttering bread. If a patient is blind or visually impaired, tell the patient what food is on the plate by comparing the plate to a clock.

For example, say, "Swiss steak is at 12 o'clock, peas and carrots are at 4 o'clock, and mashed potatoes are at 9 o'clock." Make sure all food and utensils are conveniently placed.

Before feeding any patient, test the temperature of all hot foods. A small amount can be placed on your wrist to check temperature. Never blow on hot food to cool it.

Points to observe when feeding a patient include:

- Alternate the foods by giving sips of liquids between solid foods.

- Use straws for liquids unless the patient has *dysphagia* (difficulty in swallowing). Straws can force liquids down the throat faster and cause choking. A product called Thick-It can be added to liquids to solidify them slightly and make them easier to swallow. A physician or dietitian must approve the use of this product.

- Hold the spoon or fork at right angles to the patient's mouth so you are feeding the patient from the tip of the utensil.

- Encourage the patient to eat as much as possible.

- Provide a relaxed, unhurried atmosphere.

- Give the patient sufficient time to chew the food.

Observe how much the patient eats so that a record of nutritional intake can be kept. If the patient does not like certain foods on the tray, ask your immediate supervisor or the dietitian whether a substitute can be provided.

CAUTION: Always be alert to signs of choking while feeding a patient. Take every effort to prevent choking by feeding small quantities, allowing the patient time to chew and swallow, and providing liquids to keep the mouth moist and make chewing and swallowing easier. If a patient had a stroke, one side of the mouth may be affected. As you feed the patient, direct food to the unaffected side. Watch the patient's throat to check swallowing. Watch for food that may be lodged in the affected side of the mouth. If a patient chokes on food, be prepared to provide abdominal thrusts (Heimlich maneuver) as described in Procedures 13:2D and 13:2E, CPR for Obstructed Airway in Conscious and Unconscious Victims.

STUDENT: *Complete the assignment sheet for 4:11, Feeding a Patient. Then continue with the procedure.*

4:11 FEEDING A PATIENT

ASSIGNMENT SHEET

Grade _____ Name _____

INTRODUCTION: Since good nutrition is an important part of a patient's treatment, this sheet will help you review the main facts on feeding a patient.

INSTRUCTIONS: Read the information on Feeding a Patient. In the space provided, print the word(s) that best completes the statement or answers the question.

1. List four (4) things you should do to prepare a patient for mealtime.

2. What should you do if a patient's meal will be delayed because of X-rays or other treatments?

3. If you question an item on a patient's tray (example: salt on a low-salt diet), what should you do?

4. If a patient does not like a particular food, what should you do?

5. List two (2) things you should check on the patient's tray.

6. Mr. Mendez is blind but must be encouraged to feed himself. How can you assist?

7. How can you test hot foods or liquids before feeding them to a patient?

8. Identify two (2) principles that should be followed while feeding a patient.

9. Identify two (2) ways to prevent the patient from choking while being fed.

PROCEDURE 4:11 FEEDING A PATIENT

Equipment and Supplies

Food tray with diet card, flex straws, towel, pen or pencil

Procedure

1. Obtain proper authorization and assemble equipment.

2. Knock on the door and pause before entering. Introduce yourself. Identify the patient. Explain that it is almost time to eat. Close the door and screen the unit to provide privacy.

3. Wash hands. Put on gloves if contact with oral fluids is possible.

4. Prepare the patient for mealtime. Provide oral hygiene, if desired. Help the patient use the bedpan, as needed. Position the patient in a sitting position, if permitted. Allow the patient to wash his or her hands and face. Position the overbed table.

   NOTE: Make sure the patient is not scheduled for X-ray or any other treatment requiring the tray to be withheld.

5. Check the tray. Make sure the diet card, patient's name, and food are correct. Do not add anything to the tray without first checking with your supervisor.

   NOTE: If any foods seem to be incorrect for the diet ordered, check immediately with your supervisor.

6. Place the tray on the overbed table. Place a towel or napkin under the patient's chin.

7. If the patient can feed him- or herself, arrange all food and silverware conveniently. Cut meat, butter bread, and open beverage cartons.

8. To feed a patient, proceed as follows:

   a. Follow the patient's preference for the order of foods eaten.

   b. Test hot liquids on your wrist before giving them to the patient. Wipe away any food placed on your wrist.

   c. Use drinking straws for liquids unless the patient has dysphagia. Use a separate straw for each liquid offered. Give the patient a drink of water to wet the palate and make swallowing easier.

   d. Hold utensils at a right angle (90°) to the patient's mouth. Feed the patient from the tip of the utensil.

   e. Place a small amount of food on the utensil. Fill the spoon or fork about one-third to one-half full.

   f. Tell the patient what he or she is eating.

   g. If the patient had a stroke, place food in the unaffected side of the mouth. Watch the throat to make sure the patient is swallowing.

   h. Allow time for the patient to chew. Do not hurry the patient.

   i. Alternate foods, but don't mix foods together. Provide liquids at intervals to keep the mouth moist and make chewing and swallowing easier.

   j. Allow the patient to hold bread and to help to the extent that he or she is able.

   k. Use a towel or napkin to wipe the patient's mouth, as necessary.

   ! CAUTION: Be alert at all times to signs of dysphagia and/or choking.

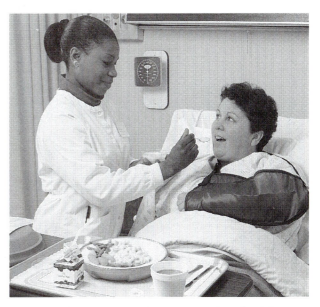

Hold utensils at a right angle to the mouth to feed the patient from the tip of the utensil.

Procedure 4:11 (cont.)

9. Encourage the patient to eat as much as possible.

   NOTE: If the patient does not like a particular food, check with your immediate supervisor or the dietitian about substitute foods.

10. When the meal is complete, allow the patient to wash his or her hands. Provide oral hygiene. Position the patient comfortably and in correct body alignment.

11. Observe all checkpoints before leaving the patient: elevate the siderails, if indicated; lower the bed to its lowest level; place the call signal and supplies within easy reach of the patient; leave the area neat and clean.

12. Note how much food was eaten.

13. Clean and replace all equipment. Place the tray in the correct area.

14. Wash hands.

15. Report that the patient has been fed and/or record all required information on the patient's chart or the agency form, for example, date; time; fed breakfast, ate everything except one-half slice toast; and your signature and title.

Practice *Use the evaluation sheet for 4:11, Feeding a Patient, to practice this procedure. When you feel you have mastered this skill, sign the sheet and give it to your instructor for further action.*

✔ **Final Checkpoint** Using the criteria listed on the evaluation sheet, your instructor will grade your performance.

Name _____ Date _____

Evaluated by _____

DIRECTIONS: Practice feeding a patient according to the criteria listed. When you are ready for your final check, give this sheet to your instructor.

Feeding a Patient	Points Possible	Yes	No	Points Earned	Comments
1. Checks orders or obtains authorization	2				
2. Assembles equipment and supplies	2				
3. Knocks on door, introduces self, identifies patient, and explains procedure	2				
4. Washes hands and puts on gloves if needed	2				
5. Prepares patient for meal:					
Provides oral hygiene if desired	2				
Offers bedpan	2				
Washes hands and face	2				
Places in sitting position	2				
Clears and positions overbed table	2				
6. Checks tray:					
Notes patient's name	2				
Checks type diet	2				
Checks foods present	2				
Substitutes or removes food only after checking	2				
7. Places tray on overbed table	2				
8. Positions napkin/towel under patient's chin	2				
9. Assists patient as needed:					
Cuts meat, butters bread	2				
Opens cartons	2				
Arranges conveniently	2				
10. Tests hot liquids or foods on wrist	4				
11. Uses separate straw for each liquid	4				
12. Holds utensil at right angle	4				
13. Feeds patient from tip of utensil	4				
14. Places small amounts on utensil	4				
15. Tells patient what he/she is eating	4				

Evaluation 4:11 (cont.)

Feeding a Patient	Points Possible	Yes	No	Points Earned	Comments
16. Provides time to chew	4				
17. Alternates solids and liquids	4				
18. Wipes mouth properly	4				
19. Encourages patient to eat as much as possible	4				
20. Watches patient closely to make sure patient is swallowing	4				
21. Allows patient to wash hands when done	3				
22. Provides oral hygiene	3				
23. Observes following checks before leaving patient:					
Patient in alignment	1				
Siderails elevated if indicated	1				
Bed at lowest level	1				
Call signal and supplies in reach	1				
Area neat and clean	1				
24. Notes and records amount of food patient ate	3				
25. Cleans and replaces all equipment	2				
26. Removes gloves if worn and washes hands	2				
27. Records or reports required information	2				
Totals	100				

OBRA Many patients require aids, or assistive devices, when ambulating. The type used depends on the injury and the patient's condition. However, certain points must be observed when a patient uses crutches.

Crutches

Crutches are artificial supports that assist a patient who needs help walking. Crutches are usually prescribed by a physician. A therapist or other authorized individual fits the crutches to the patient and teaches the appropriate gait. In addition, exercises to strengthen the muscles of the shoulders, arms, and hands are frequently prescribed by the physician or therapist. Health care workers should be aware of the criteria for fitting and of the gaits so that they can properly ambulate patients.

There are three main types of crutches:

- *Axillary crutches:* Made of wood or aluminum and used for patients who need crutches for a short period of time. The patient must be taught to bear weight on the hand bars instead of the axillary (armpit) supports. If pressure is applied on the axillary bar, it can injure axillary blood vessels and nerves. They are *not* recommended for weak or elderly patients because axillary crutches require good upper body and arm strength and a good sense of balance and coordination.

- *Forearm or Lofstrand crutches:* Attach to forearms; used for patients with weakness or paralysis in both legs; recommended for patients who need crutches permanently or for a long period of time; require upper arm strength and good coordination.

- *Platform crutches:* Used for patients who cannot grip handles of other crutches or bear weight on wrist and hands; do not require as much upper body strength, but do require a good sense of balance and coordination; require that elbows be flexed at 90° or right angle so patient can bear weight on forearm.

The following points should be observed when fitting crutches to a patient.

- The patient should wear walking shoes that fit well and provide good support. The shoes should have low, broad heels approximately 1 to 1½ inches high and nonskid soles.

- The crutches should be positioned 4 to 6 inches in front of and 4 to 6 inches to the side of the patient's foot.

- The length of axillary crutches should be adjusted so that there are 2 inches between the armpit and the axillary bar of the crutch.

- The handpieces of axillary or forearm crutches should be adjusted so that each elbow is flexed at a 25° to 30° angle.

Some of the more common crutch-walking gaits are described. The gait taught by the therapist or authorized person depends on the injury and the patient's condition.

- *Four-point gait:* Used when both legs can bear some weight. It is a slow gait. Patients often are taught the four-point gait as the first gait and are then taught faster gaits when this one is mastered.

- *Two-point gait:* Often taught after the four-point gait is mastered. It is a faster gait and is usually used when both legs can bear some weight. The two-point gait is closest to the natural rhythm of walking.

- *Three-point gait:* Used when only one leg can bear weight. It too is a gait taught initially.

- *Swing-to gait:* This is a more rapid gait. It is taught after other gaits are mastered, in most

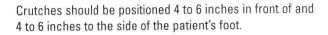

Crutches should be positioned 4 to 6 inches in front of and 4 to 6 inches to the side of the patient's foot.

cases. It requires that the patient have more shoulder and arm strength.

- *Swing-through gait:* This is the most rapid gait. However, it requires the most strength and skill. It is usually taught as a more advanced method of crutch walking.

Ambulation Precautions

CAUTION: It is essential that the health care worker remain alert at all times when ambulating a patient. Always walk on the patient's weak side and slightly behind the patient, and be alert for signs that the patient may fall. If the patient starts to fall, do *not* try to hold the patient in an upright position. Use your body to brace the patient, if at all possible: keep your back straight, bend from the hips and knees, maintain a broad base of support, and try to grasp the patient under the axillary (armpit) areas. The patient should be eased to the floor as slowly as possible. The patient's head and neck should be protected, and the head should be prevented from striking the floor. Stay with the patient and call for help. Patients should not be moved until they have been examined for injuries. After a fall has occurred, most agencies require a written incident report. Follow agency policy for correct documentation of the incident.

STUDENT: *Complete the assignment sheet for 4:12, Ambulating a Patient with Crutches. Then return and continue with the procedure.*

4:12 AMBULATING A PATIENT WITH CRUTCHES

ASSIGNMENT SHEET

Grade _____ Name _____

INTRODUCTION: This assignment sheet will help you review the main facts on crutches.

INSTRUCTIONS: Review the information on Ambulating a Patient with Crutches. In the space provided, print the word(s) that best completes the statement or answers the question.

1. When a patient is being fitted for crutches, the following measurement points should be noted:

   Height of heels on shoes: _____

   Position crutches: _____ inches to the side and front of the patient's foot.

   Distance between axilla and axillary bar: _____

   Degree angle for elbows: _____

2. If a patient can bear weight on both legs, the _____ gait is usually taught first. When the patient has mastered this gait, the _____ gait is taught next. After the patient gains strength in the arms and shoulders, faster gaits such as the _____ or _____ are taught last.

3. If a patient can bear weight on only one leg, the first crutch gait taught is the _____. When the patient gains strength in the arms and shoulders, faster gaits such as the _____ or _____ are taught.

4. Why is it important to avoid pressure on the axillary area when fitting a patient for crutches?

5. Identify the type of crutches:
   a. used for patients who need crutches for a short period of time
   b. used for patients who cannot grip handles of other crutches
   c. crutches that attach to forearms and are used by patients with paralysis of both legs

6. What should you do if a patient starts to fall while ambulating with crutches?

PROCEDURE 4:12 AMBULATING A PATIENT WITH CRUTCHES

Equipment and Supplies

Adjustable crutches, pen or pencil

Procedure

1. Check orders or obtain authorization from your immediate supervisor. Find out which gait the therapist taught the patient.

2. Assemble equipment.

3. Check the crutches. Make sure there are rubber-suction tips on the bottom ends and that the tips are not worn down or torn. Check to be sure the axillary bars and hand rests are covered with padding.
   NOTE: Foam-rubber pads are usually placed on crutches.

4. Knock on the door and pause before entering. Introduce yourself. Identify the patient. Explain the procedure.

5. Wash hands.

6. Help the patient put on good walking shoes. The shoes should have low, broad heels approximately 1 to 1½ inches high and nonskid soles.

7. Assist the patient to a standing position. Advise the patient to bear his or her weight on the unaffected leg. Position the crutches correctly.

8. Check the fit of the crutches.
   a. Position the crutches 4 to 6 inches in front of the patient's feet.
   b. Move the crutches 4 to 6 inches to the sides of the feet.
   c. Make sure there is a 2-inch gap between the axilla (armpit) and the axillary bar or rest. If the length must be adjusted, check with your immediate supervisor.
   d. Each elbow must be flexed at a 25° to 30° angle. If the hand rests must be adjusted to achieve this angle, check with your immediate supervisor.
   NOTE: In some agencies, the trained health care worker is permitted to adjust the crutches as necessary. The adjustments are then checked by the therapist or other authorized person. Follow your agency's policy.

9. Assist the patient with the required gait. The gait used depends on the patient's injury and condition. It is determined by the therapist or other authorized person.
   CAUTION: Remain alert at all times. Be ready to catch the patient if there are any signs of falling.

10. Four-point gait:
    a. The patient can bear weight on both legs. Start the patient in a standing position, with crutches at the sides.
    b. Move the right crutch forward.
    c. Move the left foot forward.
    d. Move the left crutch forward.
    e. Move the right foot forward.
    NOTE: This is a slow gait taught initially when both legs can bear weight.

11. Three-point gait:
    a. The patient can bear weight on one leg only. Start the patient in a standing position, with crutches at the sides.
    b. Advance both crutches and the weak or affected foot.

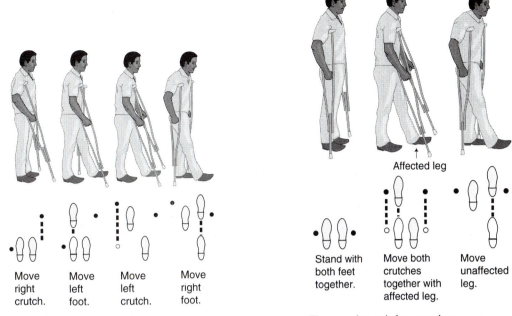

Four-point gait for crutches.

Move right crutch.   Move left foot.   Move left crutch.   Move right foot.

Three-point gait for crutches.

Stand with both feet together.   Move both crutches together with affected leg.   Move unaffected leg.

Affected leg

   c. Transfer the patient's body weight forward to the crutches.

   d. Advance the unaffected, or good, foot forward.

NOTE: This is a slow gait taught initially when only one leg can bear weight.

12. Two-point gait:

   a. The patient can bear weight on both legs. Start with the crutches at the sides.

   b. Move the right foot and left crutch forward at the same time.

   c. Move the left foot and right crutch forward at the same time.

NOTE: This is a more advanced and a more rapid gait used when the four-point gait has been mastered.

13. Swing-to gait:

   a. One or both of the patient's legs can bear weight. Start with the crutches at the sides.

   b. Balance weight on foot or feet. Move both crutches forward.

   c. Transfer weight forward.

   d. Use shoulder and arm strength to swing feet up to crutches.

NOTE: This is a more rapid gait and requires more shoulder and arm strength and a good sense of balance and coordination.

14. Swing-through gait:

   a. One or both of the patient's legs can bear weight. Start with the crutches at the sides. Balance weight on foot or feet.

   b. Advance both crutches forward at the same time.

   c. Transfer weight forward.

   d. Use shoulder and arm strength to swing up to and through the crutches, stopping slightly in front of the crutches.

NOTE: This is the most rapid and advanced gait. It requires a great deal of shoulder and arm strength. It also requires an excellent sense of balance because at one point only the crutches are in contact with the ground.

Procedure 4:12 (cont.)

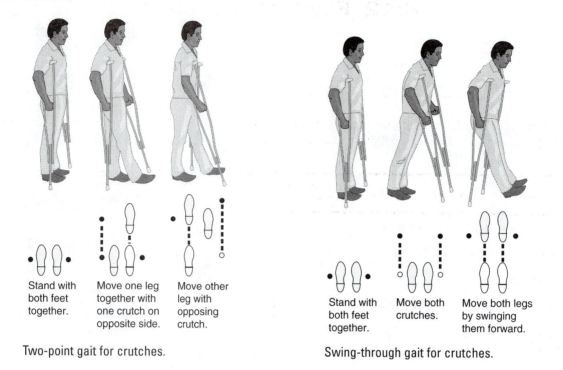

Stand with both feet together.

Move one leg together with one crutch on opposite side.

Move other leg with opposing crutch.

Two-point gait for crutches.

Stand with both feet together.

Move both crutches.

Move both legs by swinging them forward.

Swing-through gait for crutches.

15. When using crutches, the patient must *not* rest his or her body weight on the axillary rests. Shoulder and arm strength should provide movement on the crutches.

> **CAUTION:** Warn the patient that nerve damage can occur if weight is supported constantly on the axillary rest.

16. Check to make sure that the patient is not moving too far forward at one time. Distances should be limited. If the patient attempts to move the crutches too far forward, he or she can very easily lose balance and fall forward.

17. Check the patient's progress. Report the progress to the therapist or your immediate supervisor. The therapist will determine when to teach the patient more advanced gaits.

18. When the patient is finished using the crutches, replace all equipment.

19. Assist the patient back to bed or position the patient in a chair. Observe all checkpoints before leaving the patient. Make sure the patient is comfortable and in good body alignment. If the patient is in bed, elevate the siderails (if indicated), lower the bed to its lowest level, place the call signal and other supplies within easy reach of the patient, and leave the area neat and clean.

20. Wash hands.

21. Report and/or record all required information on the patient's chart or the agency form, for example, date; time; ambulated with crutches, walked down the hall two times using two-point gait, no problems noted; and your signature and title. Report any problems immediately.

Practice *Use the evaluation sheet for 4:12, Ambulating a Patient With Crutches, to practice this procedure. When you feel you have mastered this skill, sign the sheet and give it to your instructor for further action.*

✔ **Final Checkpoint** Using the criteria listed on the evaluation sheet, your instructor will grade your performance.

4:12 EVALUATION SHEET

Name _____ Date _____

Evaluated by _____

DIRECTIONS: Practice ambulating a patient with crutches according to the criteria listed. When you are ready for your final check, give this sheet to your instructor.

Ambulating a Patient with Crutches	Points Possible	Yes	No	Points Earned	Comments
1. Checks order or obtains authorization	3				
2. Assembles equipment and supplies	2				
3. Checks rubber tips on ends	3				
4. Checks padding on axillary bar and handrest	3				
5. Introduces self, identifies patient, and explains procedure	3				
6. Washes hands	2				
7. Assists patient to put on shoes:					
Low broad heel	2				
Heel 1 to 1½ inches high	2				
Nonskid soles	2				
8. Assists patient to standing position and positions crutches	3				
9. Checks measurement of crutches for following:					
Crutches 4 to 6 inches in front of feet	2				
Crutches 4 to 6 inches to side of feet	2				
2 inch gap between axilla and bar	2				
Elbow flexed at 25°–30° angle	2				
10. Assists with 4-point gait					
Moves right crutch forward	3				
Moves left foot forward	3				
Moves left crutch forward	3				
Moves right foot forward	3				
11. Assists with 3-point gait:					
Advances both crutches and affected foot	3				
Transfers body weight forward to crutches	3				
Advances unaffected foot	3				
12. Assists with 2-point gait:					
Moves right foot and left crutch forward together	4				
Moves left foot and right crutch forward together	4				

Ambulating a Patient with Crutches	Points Possible	Yes	No	Points Earned	Comments
13. Assists with swing to gait:					
Balances weight on foot/feet	3				
Moves both crutches forward	3				
Transfers weight forward	3				
Swings feet up to crutches	3				
14. Assists with swing-through gait:					
Balances weight on foot/feet	2				
Advances both crutches	2				
Transfers weight forward	2				
Swings feet up to and through crutches	2				
Stops slightly in front of crutches	2				
15. Checks that patient does not rest weight on axillary rest or bar	3				
16. Limits distances so patient not moving too far at one time	3				
17. Positions patient comfortably and observes safety checks when ambulation complete	3				
18. Replaces equipment	2				
19. Washes hands	2				
20. Records or reports required information	3				
Totals	100				

4:13 APPLYING A MOIST COMPRESS

As a veterinary worker, you may be responsible for administering a variety of heat and cold applications. Some of the main principles involved are described in this section.

Cold applications (cryotherapy) are administered to relieve pain, reduce swelling, reduce body temperature, and control bleeding.

■ **Moist cold** applications are cold and moist or wet against the skin. Examples are cold compresses, packs, and soaks. These applications are more penetrating than are dry cold applications.

■ **Dry cold** applications are cold and dry against the skin. Examples are ice bags or ice collars.

Heat applications (thermotherapy) are administered to relieve pain, increase drainage from an infected area, stimulate healing, increase circulation to an area, combat infection, and relieve muscle spasms or increase muscle mobility before exercise.

■ **Moist heat** applications are warm and wet against the skin. These applications are more penetrating and more effective in relieving pain in deeper tissues than are dry heat applications. Examples are hot soaks and compresses.

■ **Dry heat** applications are warm and dry against the skin. Examples are warm-water bags, heating pads, and heat lamps.

Heat and cold applications are effective because of the reactions they cause in the blood vessels.

■ Heat applications cause **vasodilation**. The blood vessels in the area become larger (dilated). More blood comes to the area. Therefore, more oxygen and nutrients are available to stimulate healing. Heat applications ease pain by allowing the blood to carry away fluids that cause inflammation and pain.

■ Cold applications cause **vasoconstriction**. The blood vessels become smaller (constricted). Less blood comes to the area. Swelling decreases because fewer fluids are present. The cold also has a numbing effect, which decreases local pain.

A veterinarian's order is required for a heat or cold application. The order should state the type of application, duration of treatment, temperature (if not standard), and area of application. In some states and agencies, veterinary care assistants are not allowed to administer heat or cold applications. It is important to check your agency's policy and be aware of your legal responsibilities.

Moist compresses can provide heat or cold. If a warm compress is ordered, the gauze or cloth used for the compress is placed in a basin of water warmed to a temperature of 100° to 105°F, or 37.8° to 41°C. If a cold compress is ordered, the gauze or cloth is placed in a basin filled with cold water or ice cubes or both. It is important to check the temperature of the water with a thermometer so it is accurate. An animal can be burned by a compress that is too hot.

The animal must be watched closely while a compress is in place. At times, it is necessary to used a bandage to hold the compress in position for the required amount of time. Talk to the animal softly to encourage the animal to relax. Animals become frightened just as people do. Constant reassurance and gentle care usually have a calming effect. If the animal's owner is present during the treatment, the owner can also talk to the animal to reassure it.

Standard precautions (discussed in Chapter 11:3) must be observed if any contact with blood, body fluids, secretions, or excretions is possible. An example is a moist heat application placed on a draining wound. Gloves must be worn. Hands must be washed frequently and are always washed immediately after removing gloves. A mask and eye protection must be worn if splashing or spraying of body fluids is possible. A veterinary care worker must always use proper precautions to prevent the spread of infection.

STUDENT: *Complete the assignment sheet for 4:13 Applying a Moist Compress. Then continue with the procedure.*

4:13 APPLYING A MOIST COMPRESS

ASSIGNMENT SHEET

Grade _____ Name _____

INTRODUCTION: This sheet will help you review the main facts regarding moist compresses.

INSTRUCTIONS: Review the information on Applying a Moist Compress. In the space provided, print the word(s) that best completes the statement or answers the question.

1. Define *cryotherapy*.

2. Define *thermotherapy*.

3. How do blood vessels react when heat applications are applied?

    How does this reaction affect the blood supply to the area?

4. How do blood vessels react when cold applications are applied?

    How does this reaction affect the blood supply to the area?

5. List three (3) reasons why cold applications are done.

6. List three (3) reasons why heat applications are done.

7. Define the following words, and list an example for each type of application.
    a. moist cold:
    b. dry cold:
    c. moist heat:
    d. dry heat:

8. What is the normal temperature for a warm compress?

PROCEDURE 4:13 APPLYING A MOIST COMPRESS

Equipment and Supplies

Basin; bath thermometer; underpads; washcloth, towel, or gauze pads (for compress); bath towel; plastic sheet; pen or pencil

Procedure

1. Check veterinarian's orders or obtain authorization from your immediate supervisor for the application.

2. Assemble equipment.

3. Check to be sure you have the correct animal. If the animal is in a veterinary hospital, the cages are usually marked with the animal's and owner's names. If the owner is with the animal, explain the procedure to the owner. Ask the animal's owner to assist by talking to the animal to keep it calm.

4. Wash hands. Put on gloves.

   CAUTION: Observe standard precautions if any contact with blood or body fluids is likely, such as when a compress is applied to a draining wound.

5. Position the animal in a comfortable position if possible. The position depends on the area being treated. At times, the treatment is performed while the animal is in its cage. At other times, the animal is placed on an examining table. If the animal is on an examining table, someone must be with the animal at all times to keep him or her from falling or jumping off the table.

6. Expose the area to be treated. Position an underpad near the area to be treated. This will keep the examining table clean and dry.

7. Fill the basin with water at the correct temperature. Use the bath thermometer to check the temperature.
   a. If a cold compress is to be applied, fill the basin with cold water. Ice cubes are sometimes added to the water. Do not add ice cubes unless you are told to do so.
   b. If a hot compress is to be applied, fill the basin with water at a temperature of 100° to 105°F, or 37.8° to 41°C.
   NOTE: Temperatures may vary. Follow veterinarian's orders or agency policy.

8. Put the compress (washcloth, towel, or gauze pad) in the water. Wring out the compress to remove excess liquid.

9. Apply the compress to the correct area. Use a plastic sheet to cover the area. Then wrap a bath towel around the treated area.

   NOTE: The plastic sheet helps keep the compress moist and hot or cold.

10. An ice bag or aquamatic pad is sometimes placed over the compress to help maintain the temperature. Follow agency policy or veterinarian's orders.

11. Check the compress at frequent intervals. Change the compress and remoisten it as necessary. Check the condition of the skin under the compress. If the skin is discolored, remove the compress immediately and inform your immediate supervisor.

12. Continue the treatment for the ordered period of time. Most compresses are left in place for 15 to 20 minutes.

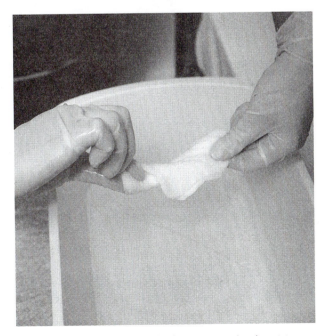

After putting the compress in the water, wring it out to remove excess liquid.

Procedure 4:13 (cont.)

13. When the ordered time has elapsed, remove the compress. Note the condition of the skin.

14. Make sure the animal has been returned to its cage or its owner. Never allow the animal to stay on the examining table if no one is present to watch it.

15. Clean and replace all equipment used. Discard gauze pads used as compresses. Place linen in a hamper or the laundry area.

16. Remove gloves. Wash hands.

17. Report and/or record all required information on the animal's chart or the agency form, for example, date; time; cold moist compresses applied to right paw for 20 minutes, no change in skin color noted; and your signature and title. Report any unusual observations immediately.

Practice *Use the evaluation sheet for 4:13, Applying a Moist Compress, to practice this procedure. When you feel you have mastered this skill, sign the sheet and give it to your instructor for further action.*

✔ **Final Checkpoint** Using the criteria listed on the evaluation sheet, your instructor will grade your performance.

Name _____ Date _____

Evaluated by _____

DIRECTIONS: Practice applying a moist compress according to the criteria listed. When you are ready for your final check, give this sheet to your instructor.

Applying a Moist Compress	Points Possible	Yes	No	Points Earned	Comments
1. Checks order or obtains authorization	4				
2. Assembles equipment and supplies	2				
3. Checks to be sure he/she has correct animal	2				
4. Positions animal and exposes area to be treated	2				
5. Washes hands and puts on gloves if necessary	3				
6. Positions underpad by area to be treated	4				
7. Fills basin with correct temperature water:					
Checks temperature with bath thermometer	4				
Uses cold water and at times ice cubes for cold compress	4				
Uses 100°–105°F or 37.8°–41°C for hot compress	4				
8. Puts compress in water	5				
9. Wrings out compress to remove excess water	5				
10. Applies compress to correct area	5				
11. Covers compress with plastic sheet and towel or underpad	5				
12. Covers with ice bag/aquamatic pad if indicated	4				
13. Removes gloves if worn and washes hands before leaving room	3				
14. Does not leave animal unattended on examining table	3				
15. Checks compress at frequent intervals:					
Changes compress and remoistens as necessary	4				
Checks condition of skin	4				
Notes pain, extreme redness	4				
Removes immediately if signs of burn present	4				

Applying a Moist Compress	Points Possible	Yes	No	Points Earned	Comments
16. Removes application at end of ordered time period	5				
17. Checks skin carefully	5				
18. Makes sure animal is back in cage or with owner before leaving	5				
19. Replaces all equipment and leaves area neat and clean	3				
20. Removes gloves if worn and washes hands	3				
21. Records or reports all required information	4				
Totals	100				

4:14 SCREENING FOR VISION PROBLEMS

Vision screening tests are often given as part of a physical examination or to detect eye disease. One method involves the use of **Snellen charts**. Snellen charts are used to test distant vision. They come in a variety of types. Some contain pictures for use with small children. Some contain the letter *E* in a variety of positions. The patient points in the direction that the *E* points. This type of chart is used for non-English-speaking people or nonreaders. Some contain letters of the alphabet. It is important to make sure the patient knows all the letters of the alphabet when using this type of chart.

Characters (that is, letters or pictures) on the Snellen chart have specific heights, ranging from small, on the bottom of the chart, to large, on the top of the chart. When standing 20 feet from the chart, a person with so-called normal vision should be able to see characters that are 20 millimeters high. Such a person is said to have 20/20 vision. In reference to 20/20 vision, the top number represents the distance the patient is from the chart. For this screening test, then, the patient is placed 20 feet from the chart. The bottom number represents the height of the characters that the patient can read at that distance.

- *Example 1:* If a patient has 20/30 vision, this means that when standing 20 feet from the chart, the patient can see characters 30 millimeters high. It can also be stated that this patient, who is standing 20 feet from the chart, can see what a patient with normal vision can see standing 30 feet from the chart.

- *Example 2:* If a patient has 20/100 vision, this means that when standing 20 feet from the chart, the patient can only see characters that are 100 mm high. This finding represents a defect in distant vision. A person with normal vision would be able to see the same figures while standing 100 feet from the chart.

It is important to note that Snellen charts test only for defects in distant vision or nearsightedness (myopia). Defects in close vision (problems with reading small print and seeing up close), known as farsightedness (hyperopia), are tested by using a printed book or cards in which the characters are certain heights. The patient holds the book or cards approximately 14 to 16 inches away from the eyes. The patient then reads printed text or identifies pictures that gradually become smaller. The smallest print or character that the patient can read or identify without error is recorded.

When screening for vision problems, there are some special terms or abbreviations to remember:

- **OD:** abbreviation for *oculus dexter*, or right eye.
- **OS:** abbreviation for *oculus sinister*, or left eye.
- **OU:** abbreviation for oculus uterque, or each eye; both eyes.
- **myopia:** nearsightedness, defect in distant vision.
- **hyperopia:** farsightedness, defect in close vision.
- **ophthalmoscope:** instrument for checking the eye.
- **tonometer:** instrument to measure intraocular tension or pressure; increased pressure often indicates glaucoma.

STUDENT: *Complete the assignment sheet for 4:14, Screening for Vision Problems. Then continue with the procedure.*

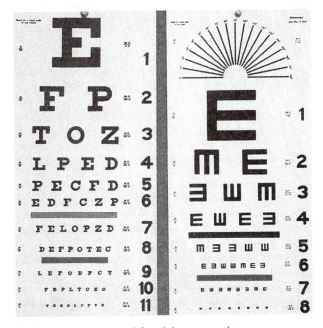

Snellen charts are used for vision screening.

4:14 SCREENING FOR VISION PROBLEMS

ASSIGNMENT SHEET

Grade _____ Name _____

INTRODUCTION: As an assistant, you may be required to screen vision with a Snellen chart. This assignment will help you review the main facts.

INSTRUCTIONS: Review the information on Screening for Vision Problems. In the space provided, print the word(s) that best completes the statement or answers the question.

1. Name three (3) types of Snellen charts.

2. Characters on the Snellen chart have specific _____, which progress from small to large figures. A patient with normal vision should be able to see figures _____ millimeters high while standing _____ feet from the chart.

3. When referring to 20/20 vision, what does the top number represent?

4. When referring to 20/20 vision, what does the bottom number represent?

5. If a patient has 20/50 vision, this means that the patient can see figures _____ millimeters high while standing _____ feet from the chart. A person with normal vision could see the same figures while standing _____ feet from the chart.

6. What vision defect is tested with the Snellen chart?

7. List the meaning of the following abbreviations.

   OD:

   OS:

   OU:

8. What is myopia?

9. What is hyperopia?

10. What is an ophthalmoscope?

PROCEDURE 4:14 SCREENING FOR VISION PROBLEMS

Equipment and Supplies

Snellen eye chart, pointer, tape, card or eye shield, paper, pen or pencil

Procedure

1. Assemble equipment.
2. Attach the Snellen chart to the wall or place it in a lighted stand. Measure a distance of 20 feet directly away from the front of the chart. Place a piece of tape on the floor at the 20-foot mark.

   NOTE: Most medical offices will have a mark on the floor to indicate the 20-foot distance.
3. Wash hands.
4. Introduce yourself. Identify the patient. Explain the procedure.

   NOTE: If using a chart with letters, make sure the patient knows the letters of the alphabet. If using a picture chart, make sure small children know what each picture represents.
5. Instruct the patient to stand facing the chart. Make sure the patient's toes are on the taped line; the patient's eyes will be 20 feet from the chart.
6. Point to various letters or pictures on the chart. Ask the patient to identify the letters or pictures. If the patient wears corrective lenses (glasses or contact lenses), check the vision with the corrective lenses first. Then ask the patient to remove the corrective lenses. Check the vision again. Record both readings. Observe the following points:
   a. Start with the larger letters or pictures and proceed to the smaller ones.
   b. Make sure the pointer you are using does not block the letters or pictures.
   c. Select letters or pictures at random in each row. Do *not* start at one end of the row and go straight across the line. Patients may memorize order; random sampling makes the patient focus on individual letters or pictures.
      NOTE: If you are sure the patient has not memorized the letters, you may ask the patient to read a row of letters. If the patient is able to read all letters correctly, proceed to a smaller row.
   d. Watch to be sure the patient is not leaning forward or squinting to see the letters or pictures.

   NOTE: Some examiners do the left or right eye first, the opposite eye second, and both eyes last. Follow your agency's policy.
7. Ask the patient to correctly identify all the letters or pictures in the 20/20 line. If the patient is unable to do so, note the line that the patient *can* read with 100 percent accuracy.
8. Give the patient an eye shield or card with which to cover the left eye. Warn the patient not to close the left eye while it is covered, because doing so can cause blurred vision. Repeat steps 6 and 7 to test the vision in the right eye (OD).

   CAUTION: Warn the patient against pressing on the covered eye to avoid injuring the eye with the card or shield. Do *not* use the card or shield on another patient. Discard it after use.
9. Ask the patient to cover the right eye. Repeat steps 6 and 7 to test the vision in the left eye (OS).

   NOTE: Remind the patient to keep the right eye open while it is covered.
10. Record the test results for both eyes, the right eye, and the left eye. Use abbreviations of *OU*, *OD*, and *OS* and readings of *20/20*, *20/30*, or the correct reading.
11. Thank the patient for being cooperative.

    NOTE: This is a screening test only. Unfavorable results indicate the need for additional testing or referral to an eye specialist.
12. Clean and replace all equipment. If the eye shield is not disposable, wash it thoroughly and clean it with a disinfectant solution.

Procedure 4:14 (cont.)

13. Wash hands.

14. ▨ Record all required information on the patient's chart or the agency form, for example, date, time, vision screening with Snellen chart: OU 20/30, OD 20/40, OS 20/30; and your signature and title.

Practice *Use the evaluation sheet for 4:14, Screening for Vision Problems, to practice this procedure. When you feel you have mastered this skill, sign the sheet and give it to your instructor for further action.*

✔ **Final Checkpoint** Using the criteria listed on the evaluation sheet, your instructor will grade your performance.

4:14 EVALUATION SHEET

Name _____ Date _____

Evaluated by _____

DIRECTIONS: Practice screening vision according to the criteria listed. When you are ready for your final check, give this sheet to your instructor.

Screening for Vision Problems	Points Possible	Yes	No	Points Earned	Comments
1. Assembles equipment and supplies	3				
2. Positions Snellen chart	4				
3. Places tape 20 feet from chart	5				
4. Washes hands	3				
5. Introduces self, identifies patient, and explains procedure	4				
6. Tells patient to stand with toes on tape line	5				
7. Screens both eyes:					
Points to figures without blocking them	5				
Points to large figures first	5				
Selected figures at random	5				
Checks patient for squinting or leaning forward	5				
Records correct reading	5				
8. Screens right eye:					
Instructs patient on covering left eye	5				
Selects figures at random	5				
Checks patient for squinting or leaning forward	5				
Records correct reading	5				
9. Screens left eye:					
Instructs patient to cover right eye	5				
Selects figures at random	5				
Checks patient for squinting or leaning forward	5				
Records correct reading	5				
10. Dismisses patient when test complete	4				
11. Cleans and replaces all equipment and disinfects eye shield if not disposable	3				
12. Washes hands	4				
Totals	100				

CHAPTER 4 INTERNET SEARCHES

Use the suggested search engines in Chapter 9:4 of the textbook to search the Internet for additional information on the following topics:

1. *National Health Care Skill Standards (NHCSS).*

2. *Health care careers:* Search for information on specific careers by entering the name of the career.

3. *Career organizations:* Contact organizations at web addresses listed in each career cluster to determine the purpose of the organization, health careers it promotes, and advantages of membership.

4. *Accreditation agencies:* Search the Commission on Accreditation of Allied Health Education Programs (CAAHEP) at *www.caahep.org* and the Accrediting Bureau of Health Education Schools (ABHES) at www.abhes.org to determine which health career programs are accredited by each agency. Research schools in your area that meet accreditation standards.

5. *Schools:* Search for technical schools, colleges, and universities that offer educational programs for a specific career. Evaluate entrance requirements, financial aid, and programs of study.

ASSIGNMENT SHEET

Grade _____ Name _____

INTRODUCTION: All health care workers must understand the legal and ethical responsibilities of their particular health career. This assignment will help you review the basic facts on legal and ethical responsibilities.

INSTRUCTIONS: Read the information on Legal and Ethical Responsibilities. In the space provided, print the word(s) that best completes the statement or answers the question.

1. Use the Key Terms to fill in the blanks.

    a.   C _ _ _ _ _ _ _ (agreement between two or more parties)

    b.   _ O _ _ (wrongful acts that do not involve contracts)

    c.   _ _ _ N _ _ _ (spoken defamation)

    d.   _ _ F _ _ _ _ _ _ _ (a false statement that causes a person to be ridiculed)

    e.   _ I _ _ _ (written defamation)

    f.   _ _ _ _ D _ _ _ _ _ _ _ _ _ (does not have legal capacity to form a contract)

    g.   _ E _ _ _ (authorized or based on law)

    h.   _ _ _ N _ (person working under principal's direction)

    i.   _ T _ _ _ _ (principles relating to what is morally right or wrong)

    j.   _ _ _ _ _ I _ _ _ _ _ _ _ _ _ _ _ (restricting an individual's freedom)

    k.   _ _ _ _ _ A _ _ _ _ _ (bad practice)

    l.   _ _ _ _ _ L _ (threat or attempt to injure)

    m.   _ _ _ _ I _ _ _ _ _ (failure to give expected care)

    n.   _ _ _ _ _ _ T _ _ _ _ _ _ _ (factors of care patients can expect)
                           Y

2. Create a situation that provides an example that could lead to legal action for each of the following torts.

    a. malpractice:

    b. negligence:

c. assault and battery:

d. invasion of privacy:

e. false imprisonment:

f. abuse:

g. defamation:

3. How are slander and libel the same? How are they different?

4. What are the three (3) parts of a contract?

5. What is the difference between an implied and an expressed contract?

6. List three (3) examples of individuals who have legal disabilities.

7. What legal requirement must be followed when a contract is explained to a non-English-speaking individual?

8. Why is it important for a health care worker to be aware of his or her role as an agent? Who is responsible for the actions of the agent?

9. What are privileged communications?

   What must the patient do before privileged communications can be told to anyone else?

10. List three (3) examples of information that is exempt (not included) by law and not considered to be privileged communications.

11. Who owns health care records?

   What rights do patients have in regard to their health care records?

12. What should you do if you make an error while recording information on health care records?

13. List three (3) ways health care facilities create safeguards to maintain computer confidentiality.

14. What are ethics?

15. What should you do in the following situations to maintain your legal and ethical responsibilities?

   a. A patient dying of cancer tells you he has saved a supply of sleeping pills and intends to commit suicide.

   b. You work in a nursing home and see a co-worker shove a patient into a chair and then slap the patient in the face.

   c. You work as a dental assistant and a patient asks you, "Will the doctor be able to save this tooth or will it have to be pulled?"

   d. A patient has just been admitted to an assisted care facility. As you are helping the patient undress and get ready for bed, you notice numerous bruises and scratches on both arms.

16. What is the name of the act that guarantees certain rights to residents in long-term care facilities?

17. What is the purpose for each of the following advance directives for health care?

   a. Living will:

   b. Durable Power of Attorney (POA):

18. What is the purpose of the Patient Self-Determination Act (PSDA)?

19. Describe two (2) ways you can identify a patient.

20. What should you do in the following situations to maintain professional standards?

   a. The doctor you work for asks you to give a patient an allergy shot, but you are not qualified to give injections.

   b. An elderly patient, who is frequently confused and disoriented, refuses to let you take his temperature.

   c. You work in a medical laboratory. A patient's wife asks you if her husband's blood test was positive for an infectious disease.

21. What is a *DNR* order? What does DNR mean?

CHAPTER 5 INTERNET SEARCHES

Use the suggested search engines in Chapter 9:4 of the textbook to search the Internet for additional information on the following topics:

1. *Torts:* Search for additional information or actual legal cases involving malpractice, negligence, assault and battery, invasion of privacy, false imprisonment, and defamation.

2. *Abuse:* Research domestic violence or abuse, child abuse, and elder abuse to determine how victims might react, signs and symptoms that may indicate abuse, and information on how to help these victims.

3. *Contracts:* Search for information on components of a contract and legal cases in health care caused by a breach of contract.

4. *Ethics:* Use Internet addresses for professional organizations (see Chapter 4) to find two or three different codes of ethics; compare the codes of ethics.

5. *Patient's rights:* Search for complete copies of a patient's or resident's bill of rights; compare the different bills of rights (*Hint:* check American Hospital Association web site).

6. *Advance directives:* Search for different examples of a living will and/or a durable power of attorney for health care; compare the different forms.

7. *Patient Self-Determination Act of 1990:* Locate a copy of this act or information on the purposes of this act (Hint: check federal legislation web sites).

ASSIGNMENT SHEET

Grade _____ Name _____

INTRODUCTION: Every health care provider must be aware of the factors that cause each individual to be unique. This assignment will help you learn these factors.

INSTRUCTIONS: Read the information on Cultural Diversity. In the space provided, print the word(s) that best completes the statement or answers the question.

1. Define *culture*.

2. List the four (4) basic characteristics of culture.

3. A classification of people based on national origin and/or culture is _____.
   A classification of people based on physical or biological characteristics is _____.
   The differences among people resulting from cultural, ethnic, and racial factors is _____.

4. Do you think the United States is a multicultural society? Why or why not?

5. Label each of the following statements as a bias, prejudice, or stereotype.

   a. All fat people are lazy.

   b. Chemotherapy (treatment with drugs) is much better than radiation to treat cancer.

c. Herbal remedies are a waste of money.

d. All teenagers are reckless drivers.

e. He must be really stupid because he does not know how to use the Internet.

6. Identify four (4) ways to avoid bias, prejudice, and stereotyping.

7. What is holistic care?

8. Identify four (4) areas of cultural diversity.

9. Identify the following types of family organization.

   a. father is the authority figure:

   b. family consists of mother, father, and two children:

   c. parents, children, and grandparents all live in one home:

   d. mother is the authority figure:

10. Identify the culture(s) that may have the following health care beliefs.

    a. illness is caused by an imbalance between yin and yang:

    b. wearing an Azabache will treat disease:

    c. health is a balance between "hot and cold" forces:

    d. tolerating pain is a sign of strength:

    e. males make decisions on the health care of the family:

    f. shaman or medicine man is the traditional healer:

    g. health can be maintained by diet, rest, and exercise:

11. Are spirituality and religion the same? Why or why not?

12. Why is it important for a health care provider to be aware of the beliefs about death in different religions?

13. Name two (2) religions that may prohibit blood transfusions.

14. A person who does not believe in any deity is a/an _____. A person who believes the existence of God cannot be proved or disproved is a/an _____.

15. List six (6) ways to respect cultural diversity by appreciating and respecting the personal characteristics of others.

16. How would you respond to the following situations?

    a. You work as a dental assistant and attempt to explain preoperative (before surgery) instructions to a patient who is scheduled for oral surgery. He has limited English-speaking abilities and is nodding his head yes, but he does not seem to understand the instructions.

b. You work as a surgical technician and prepare a patient for surgery. When you tell her she must remove all jewelry, she says she never removes her cross necklace.

c. You work as an electrocardiograph technician, and a patient has given you permission to perform an electrocardiogram. As you start to position the electrodes for each of the leads, the patient becomes very tense, pulls his arm away, and appears anxious and very nervous.

d. You have just started working as a geriatric assistant. As you prepare to bathe a patient, she tells you that she will wait until her daughter arrives and that her daughter will help her with her bath.

CHAPTER 6 INTERNET SEARCHES

Use the suggested search engines in Chapter 9:4 of the textbook to search the Internet for additional information on the following topics:

1. *Cultural diversity:* Search words such as *culture*, *ethnicity*, and *race* to obtain additional information on characteristics and examples for each.

2. *Ethnic groups:* Search countries of origin for information on different ethnic groups or on your own ethnic group; for example, if you are German–Irish, search for information on both Germany and Ireland.

3. *Cultural assimilation and acculturation:* Search for additional information on these two topics.

4. *Bias, prejudice, and stereotyping:* Use these key words to search for more detailed information.

5. *Family structure:* Search words such as *extended family*, *nuclear family*, *patriarchal*, and *matriarchal*.

6. *Health care beliefs:* Search by country of origin for health care beliefs, or search words such as *yin and yang* or *shaman*.

7. *Alternative health care:* Search for additional information on chiropractor, homeopath, naturopath, hypnotist, hypnotherapy, meditation, biofeedback, acupuncture, acupressure, therapeutic touch, yoga, tai chi, and faith healing.

8. *Spirituality and religion:* Search for additional information on spirituality; use the name of a religion to obtain more information about the beliefs and practices of the religion.

CHAPTER 7 MEDICAL TERMINOLOGY

7:1 USING MEDICAL ABBREVIATIONS

ASSIGNMENT SHEET

Grade _____ Name _____

INTRODUCTION: Shortened forms of words (often just letters) are called abbreviations. You are probably familiar with some such as AM, which means morning, and PM, which means afternoon or evening. The world of medicine has many of its own abbreviations. At times they are used by themselves. At other times, several abbreviations are used together to give orders or directions.

As a health care worker, you will be given many directions in abbreviated form. You will be expected to know their meaning. The following assignment will assist you in starting to see how these abbreviations are used and how you must translate them to understand them.

INSTRUCTIONS: Review the information on standard medical abbreviations. Try to recall the meanings of the following terms before using the textbook to find the answers.

A. Print the meanings of the following abbreviations and symbols.

1. OR _____

2. prn _____

3. ac _____

4. stat _____

5. RN _____

6. wt _____

7. Cl _____

8. Rx _____

9. AP _____

10. T _____

11. NPO _____

12. $\overline{c}$ _____

13. $\overline{ss}$ _____

14. $\overline{s}$ _____

15. BP _____

16. R _____

17. CDC _____

18. DRG _____

19. ↑ _____

20. ♀ _____

B. Look up the meanings of the following combinations to interpret the orders. Print your answers.

1. TPR qid _____

_____

2. 2 gtts bid _____

_____

3. 1 cc IM _____

_____

4. BP q 4 h _____

_____

5. 2 oz OJ qid ac and HS _____

_____

6. Wt and Ht qod in AM _____

_____

7. BR c̄ BRP only _____

_____

8. 1000 cc N/S IV _____

_____

9. Do ECG in CCU _____

_____

10. Dissolve 2 tsp NaCl in 1 qt H_2O _____

_____

11. Schedule Bl Wk in AM including CBC, BUN, and FBS _____

_____

12. 1 cap qid pc and HS _____

_____

13. BP is measured in mm of Hg _____

_____

14. NPO pre-op _____

_____

15. Do EENT exam in OPD _____

_____

16. 500 mg qod 8 AM _____

_____

17. VS stat and q2h _____

_____

18. To PT by w/c for ROMs and ADL bid _____

_____

19. FF1 cl liq to 240 cc q2h _____

_____

20. 2 gtts OU qid q6h _____

_____

7:1 EVALUATION SHEET

Name _____ Date _____

Evaluated by _____

DIRECTIONS: Read each case history aloud, using words instead of the abbreviations. Each abbreviation has a value of 5 points.

Using Medical Abbreviations	Points Possible	Yes	No	Points Earned	Comments
1. Mary was taking medicine *ac* because the *Dr* ordered it. She was complaining of not feeling well so the orders included tests to find out the reason: a *CBC* was done and also a *FBS*. When he received the results, Dr. Pierce made a *dx* of diabetes and asked the *RN* to give Mary insulin. Mary now has to take insulin *qd* by *sc inj* and is on a low-cal diet.	45				
2. A man was brought into the *ER*, but he was *DOA*. The ambulance attendant said that the man had complained of headache, his *BP* was very high, and he may have had a *CVA*.	20				
3. John Smith was taken to the *OPD* after a fall. He had a *Fr* of the knee that required surgery. After going to the *OR*, John was given medication *prn* for pain and was scheduled for *PT* to start next week for *ROM* exercises and *ADL*.	35				
Totals	100				

7:2 INTERPRETING WORD PARTS

ASSIGNMENT SHEET

Grade _____ Name _____

INTRODUCTION: Special words used in medicine are called medical terminology. Many of these words have common beginnings (prefixes), common endings (suffixes), and common parts (word roots). By learning the main prefixes, suffixes, and word roots, you can put together many new words or break apart a medical term to understand its meaning.

In the health fields, you will be required to know and understand medical terminology. Even if you have never come into contact with a medical word before, by breaking it down into its parts, you will usually be able to figure out the meaning of the word. This assignment sheet will show you the process.

INSTRUCTIONS: Review the information sheet on prefixes, suffixes, and word roots.

Study the following examples of breaking a word into parts.

Example 1:   *erythrocyte:* erythro / cyte

erythro means red

cyte means cell

erythrocyte means red cell

Example 2:   *hyperadenosis:* hyper / aden / osis

hyper means increased

aden means gland

osis means condition, state, or process

hyperadenosis means increased glandular condition

Identifying Word Parts: Determine the meanings of the following words. Print your answers in the spaces provided. The words have been separated to help you do this exercise.

1. crani / otomy _____

   crani _____

   otomy _____

2. dys / uria _____

   dys _____

   uria _____

3. hyster / ectomy _____

   hyster _____

   ectomy _____

4. hemo / toxic _____

   hemo _____

   toxic _____

5. peri / card / itis _____

   peri _____

   card _____

   itis _____

6. leuko / cyte _____

   leuko _____

   cyte _____

7. chole / cyst / itis _____

   chole _____

   cyst _____

   itis _____

8. tachy / cardia _____

   tachy _____

   cardia _____

9. neur / algia _____

   neur _____

   algia _____

10. poly / cyt / emia _____

    poly _____

    cyt _____

    emia _____

11. brady / cardia _____

    _____

    _____

12. gastr / ectomy _____

    _____

    _____

13. mening / itis _____

    _____

    _____

14. neo / pathy _____

    _____

    _____

15. dermat / ologist _____

    _____

    _____

16. aden / oma _____

_____

_____

17. hypo / glyc / emia _____

_____

_____

18. electro / encephalo / graph _____

_____

_____

19. cyt / ologist _____

_____

_____

20. para / plegia _____

_____

_____

21. py / uria _____

_____

_____

22. angio / pathy _____

_____

_____

23. geront / ology _____

_____

_____

24. dys / phagia _____

_____

_____

25. hydro / cele _____

_____

_____

7:2 EVALUATION SHEET

Name _____ Date _____

Evaluated by _____

DIRECTIONS: Be able to tell your instructor the meaning of the *italicized words*. Pronunciation, spelling, and definition of the medical term will be evaluated. Be prepared to spell the word without looking at the term.

Interpreting Word Parts	Points Possible	Yes	No	Points Earned	Comments
1. Mary had *dermalgia* that was caused by a rash.	10				
2. Mary's friend had *phlebitis*.	10				
3. *Anuria* may be a sign of kidney disease.	10				
4. A *nephrectomy* requires a surgeon's skill.	10				
5. The *gastric* secretions were high in acid content.	10				
6. A *hysterectomy* was done to remove the tumor.	10				
7. *Hyperglycemia* may be a sign of diabetes.	10				
8. *Cholecystitis* may be caused by eating large quantities of indigestible fats.	10				
9. A fractured neck can cause *quadriplegia*.	10				
10. *Hepatitis* can produce a yellow tinge to the skin.	10				
Totals	100				

CHAPTER 7 INTERNET SEARCHES

Use the suggested search engines in Chapter 9:4 of the textbook to search the Internet for additional information on the following topics:

1. *Medical terminology resources:* Search publishers such as Delmar Learning, Mosby, or McGraw-Hill, for medical terminology books, videos, and software. Evaluate different methods of learning medical terminology as presented in these resources.

2. *Diseases:* Combine word parts to name at least two (2) diseases or conditions such as *cholecystitis.* Search for information on the diseases. Research the cause of the disease, signs and symptoms, and main forms of treatment.

3. *Cancer:* Combine word parts to create words ending in *oma.* Then search for information on at least two (2) types of tumors. (*Hint:* Locate the web site for the American Cancer Society.)

CHAPTER 8 MEDICAL MATH

ASSIGNMENT SHEET

Grade _____ Name _____

INTRODUCTION: This assignment will help you review math concerns and concepts that are essential to working in health care.

INSTRUCTIONS: Read the information on Medical Math. In the space provided, print the word(s) that best completes the statement or answers the question.

1. _____ are what we traditionally use to count, they do not contain fractions or decimals. _____ are one way of expressing parts of numbers and are expressed in units of 10. _____ have a numerator and a denominator. It is easier to calculate _____ if you first convert them to decimals. _____ show relationships between numbers or like values: how many of one number of value is present as compared with the other. _____ a number means changing it to the nearest ten, hundred, thousand, and so on.

2. List three (3) guidelines to make estimating useful.

3. Perform the calculations indicated for whole numbers.

   a. $742 + 1{,}259 =$

   b. $238{,}031 - 152{,}987 =$

   c. $22 \times 156 =$

   d. $555 \div 15 =$

4. Perform the calculations indicated for decimals.

   a. $5.893 + 87.32 + 0.5 =$

   b. $78.3 - 49.538 =$

   c. $28.561 \times 5.39 =$

   d. $125.49 \div 2.35 =$

5. Perform the calculations indicated for fractions.

   a. $1/8 + 3/4 + 1/2 =$

   b. $15/16 - 3/8 =$

   c. $7/12 \times 8/21 =$

   d. $7/8 \div 5/6 =$

6. Perform the calculations indicated for percentages.

    a. 38% + 53.5% =

    b. 54.3% − 11.4% =

    c. 230 × 5% =

    d. 563 ÷ 2% =

7. Round the following numbers to the place indicated.

    a. 9,837 to the nearest tenth =

    b. 652 to the nearest hundredth =

    c. 1,479 to the nearest thousandth =

8. Use proportions to calculate the following problems.

    a. How many 250-mg tablets must be given for a total dosage of 750 mg?

    b. How many 5-grain aspirins must be given for a total dosage of 15 grains?

    c. How many milligrams of medication should you give an 80-pound person if dosage requires 20 mg for every 10 pounds of weight?

    d. If 45 milliliters of water is required to mix 100 grams of plaster, how many milliliters would you need for 200 grams of plaster?

9. Convert the following numbers to Roman numerals.

    a. 55

    b. 109

    c. 788

    d. 2367

10. Interpret the following Roman numerals.

    a. XII

    b. CCXIX

    c. XLIV

    d. DCXCII

11. Give three (3) examples of how angles are used in health care.

12. Convert the following as indicated. Use the approximate equivalents shown in the textbook to calculate your answers.

    a. 5 teaspoons = ? milliliters

    b. 2,000 milliliters = ? quarts

    c. 33 kilograms = ? pounds

    d. 6 ounces = ? milliliters

    e. 2 feet = ? centimeters

13. Convert the following temperatures from Fahrenheit to Celsius and round off the answer to the nearest one-tenth of a degree.

    a. 35°F

    b. 72°F

14. Convert the following temperatures from Celsius to Fahrenheit and round off the answer to the nearest one-tenth of a degree.

    a. 30°C

    b. 62°C

15. Define *military time*.

16. Convert the following to military time.

    a. 1:00 PM

    b. 2:00 AM

    c. 12:00 NOON

    d. 8:35 PM

    e. 5:05 AM

    f. 12:00 MIDNIGHT

CHAPTER 8 INTERNET SEARCHES

Use the suggested search engines in Chapter 9:4 of the textbook to search the Internet for additional information on the following topics:

1. *Math:* Search words such as *math*, *basic math*, *basic calculations*, *fractions*, and *percentages*.

2. *Roman numerals:* Search for additional information on using Roman numerals.

3. *Measurement:* Search words such as *measurement*, *mass/weight*, *volume*, *converting measures*, *metric system*, and *equivalents*.

4. *Temperature:* Search for information on Fahrenheit, centigrade, Celsius, and converting temperatures.

5. *Military time:* Search words such as *time*, *military time*, and *24-hour clock*.

CHAPTER 9 COMPUTERS IN HEALTH CARE

ASSIGNMENT SHEET

Grade _____ Name _____

INTRODUCTION: The computer has become an essential ingredient in almost every aspect of health care. This assignment will help you review the main facts about computers.

INSTRUCTIONS: Read the information on Computers in Health Care. In the space provided, print the word(s) that best completes the statement or answers the question.

1. Name four (4) general areas of health care that use computers.

2. Define *computer literacy.*

3. List at least four (4) commonly used items that contain computer chips.

4. A computer system is a/an _____ device that can be thought of as a complete _____. It can _____, _____, _____, _____, _____, _____, _____, and _____ data.

5. What is the difference between hardware and software?

6. Identify at least four (4) input devices that can be used to enter data into the computer.

7. What is the function of the central processing unit (CPU) of the computer?

8. What is the difference between the read only memory (ROM) and the random access memory (RAM) in the internal memory unit of a computer?

9. What is output?

   Name two (2) output devices.

10. Health care providers use computers to perform many functions. Identify at least four (4) of these functions.

11. How can confidentiality be maintained while using a computer for patient records?

12. What advantage does computerized tomography have over regular X-rays?

13. How does ultrasonography create an image of the body part such as a developing fetus?

14. What is a major use for the Internet in health care?

15. The use of computers has introduced many new abbreviations. Identify the following abbreviations as they pertain to computers.
    a. CAI
    b. CPU
    c. CT
    d. MRI
    e. PET

CHAPTER 9 INTERNET SEARCHES

Use the suggested search engines in Chapter 9:4 of the textbook to search the Internet for additional information on the following topics:

1. *Computer hardware:* Obtain information about different computer systems and compare the systems by searching the sites of computer manufacturers such as Gateway, Dell, Compaq, and IBM.

2. *Computer software:* Search for different types of software for health care providers.

3. *Diagnostic devices:* Search for additional information on blood analyzers, echocardiographs, computerized tomography, magnetic resonance imaging, positron emission tomography, and ultrasonography.

4. *Search engines:* Search for information on the main search engines, advantages and disadvantages of the engines, and ways to use the engines most effectively.

CHAPTER 10 PROMOTION OF SAFETY

10:1 USING BODY MECHANICS

ASSIGNMENT SHEET

Grade _____ Name _____

INTRODUCTION: The correct use of body mechanics is essential to protect both the worker and the patient. This sheet will allow you to review the main facts.

INSTRUCTIONS: Review the information in the text about Using Body Mechanics. Put the text aside and answer the following questions. Print your answers in the spaces provided.

1. Define *body mechanics.*

2. List three (3) reasons for using correct body mechanics.

3. In the following diagrams, certain rules for correct body mechanics are not being observed. At least three rules are being broken in each diagram. In the space provided for each diagram, list three rules not being observed.

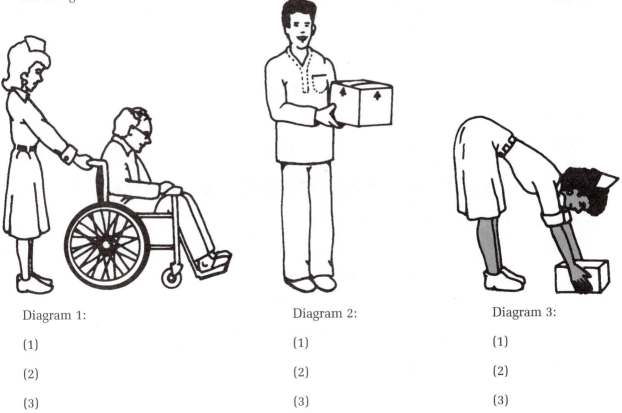

Diagram 1:

(1)

(2)

(3)

Diagram 2:

(1)

(2)

(3)

Diagram 3:

(1)

(2)

(3)

PROCEDURE 10:1 USING BODY MECHANICS

Equipment and Supplies

Heavy book, bedside stand, bed with wheel locks (**NOTE:** Two desks can be used in place of a bed and bedside stand.)

Procedure

1. Assemble equipment.

2. Compare using a narrow base of support with using a broad base of support.
   - Stand on your toes, with your feet close together.
   - Stand on your toes with your feet farther apart.
   - Stand with your feet flat on the floor but close together.
   - Stand with your feet flat on the floor but approximately 8 to 10 inches apart. Position one foot slightly forward. Balance your weight on both feet.

   You should feel the best support in the final position because the broad base supports your body weight.

3. Place the book on the floor. Bend from the hips and knees (not the waist) and keep your back straight to pick up the book. Return to the standing position.

4. Place the book between your thumb and fingers, but not touching the palm of your hand, and hold your hand straight out in front of your body. Slowly move your hand toward your body, stopping several times to feel the weight of the book in different positions. Finally, hold the book with your entire hand and bring your hand close to your body. The final position should be the most comfortable.

   NOTE: This illustrates the need to carry heavy objects close to your body and to use the strongest muscles to do the job.

5. Stand at either end of the bed. Release the wheel locks on the bed. Position your feet to provide a broad base of support. Get close to the bed. Use the weight of your body to push the bed forward.

6. Place the book on the bed. Pick up the book and place it on the bedside stand. Avoid twisting your body. Turn with your feet to place the book on the stand.

   NOTE: Remember that holding the book close to your body allows you to use the strongest muscles.

7. Practice the rules of body mechanics by setting up situations similar to those listed in the previous steps. Continue until the movements feel natural to you.

8. Replace all equipment used.

Practice *Use the evaluation sheet for 10:1, Using Body Mechanics, to practice this procedure. When you feel you have mastered this skill, sign the sheet and give it to your instructor for further action.*

✔ **Final Checkpoint** Using the criteria listed on the evaluation sheet, your instructor will grade your performance.

10:1 Evaluation Sheet

Name _____ Date _____

Evaluated by _____

DIRECTIONS: Practice body mechanics according to the criteria listed. When you are ready for your final check, give this sheet to your instructor for evaluation.

Using Body Mechanics	Points Possible	Yes	No	Points Earned	Comments
1. Demonstrates broad base of support:					
Keeps feet 8 to 10 inches apart	5				
Puts one foot slightly forward	5				
Points toes in direction of movement	5				
Balances weight on both feet	5				
2. Picks up heavy object:					
Gets close to object	6				
Maintains broad base of support	6				
Bends from hips and knees	6				
Uses strongest muscles	6				
3. Pushes heavy object:					
Gets close to object	8				
Maintains broad base of support	8				
Uses weight of body	8				
4. Carries heavy object:					
Keeps object close to body	8				
Uses strongest muscles	8				
5. Changes direction:					
Maintains broad base of support	8				
Turns with feet and entire body	8				
Totals	100				

10:2 PREVENTING ACCIDENTS AND INJURIES

ASSIGNMENT SHEET

Grade _____ Name _____

INTRODUCTION: Safety standards have been established to protect you and the patient. This sheet will help you to review the main standards.

INSTRUCTIONS: Read the information on Preventing Accidents and Injuries. In the space provided, print the word(s) that best completes the statement or answers the question.

1. What is OSHA? What is its purpose?

2. List three (3) types of information that must be included on Material Safety Data Sheets (MSDSs).

3. What is the hazardous ingredient in Clorox bleach? (*Hint:* Review the MSDS figure on Figure 10-4 in the textbook.)

4. Identify three (3) body fluids included in the bloodborne pathogen standard.

5. Name the three (3) main diseases that can be contracted by exposure to body fluids.

6. List two (2) rules or standards to observe while working with solutions in the laboratory.

7. List two (2) rules or standards to observe while working with equipment in the laboratory.

8. Before you perform any procedure on patients, there are several standards you must observe. List two (2) of these standards.

9. Identify two (2) ways to show respect for a patient's right to privacy.

10. What are two (2) methods you can use to correctly identify a patient?

11. List four (4) safety checkpoints that should be observed before leaving a patient or resident in a bed.

12. Briefly state how you should handle the following situations.

    a. You cut your hand slightly on a piece of glass:

    b. You get a particle in your eye:

    c. You turn a piece of equipment on, but it does not run properly:

    d. You spill an acid solution on the counter:

Equipment and Supplies

Information on Preventing Accidents and Injuries, several bottles of solutions, laboratory area with equipment

Procedure

1. Assemble equipment.

2. Review the safety standards in the textbook for Preventing Accidents and Injuries. Note standards that are not clear and ask your instructor for an explanation.

3. Examine several bottles of solutions. Read the labels carefully. Read the safety or danger warnings on the bottles. Read Material Safety Data Sheets provided with hazardous chemicals.

4. Practice reading the label three times to be sure you have the correct solution. Read the label before taking the bottle off the shelf, before pouring from the bottle, and after you have poured from the bottle.

5. Look at major pieces of equipment in the laboratory. Read the operating instructions for the equipment. Do *not* operate the equipment until you are taught how to do it correctly.

6. Role play the following situations by using another student as a patient.
   - Show ways to provide privacy for the patient.
   - Identify the patient.
   - Explain a procedure to the patient.
   - Check various patient areas in the laboratory. Note any safety hazards that may be present. Discuss how you can correct the problems. Report your findings to your instructor.
   - Observe the patient during a procedure. List points you should observe to note a change in the patient's condition.

7. Discuss the following situations with another student and decide how you would handle them:
   - You see an unsafe situation or a violation of a safety practice.
   - You see a wet area on the laboratory counter.
   - You get a small cut on your hand while using a glass slide.
   - A solution splashes on your arm.
   - A particle gets in your eye.
   - A piece of equipment is not working properly.
   - A bottle of solution does not have a label.
   - You break a glass thermometer.

8. Observe and practice all of the safety regulations as you work in the laboratory.

9. Study the regulations in preparation for the safety examination. You must pass the safety examination.

10. Replace all equipment used.

Practice *Use the evaluation sheet for 10:2, Preventing Accidents and Injuries, to practice this procedure. When you feel you have mastered this skill, sign the sheet and give it to your instructor for further action.*

✔ **Final Checkpoint** Using the criteria listed on the evaluation sheet, your instructor will grade your performance.

10:2 EVALUATION SHEET

Name _____ Date _____

Evaluated by _____

DIRECTIONS: Practice safety according to the criteria listed. When you are ready for your final check, give this sheet to your instructor. Given simulated situations and using the proper equipment and supplies, you will be expected to respond orally or demonstrate the following safety criteria.

Preventing Accidents and Injuries	Points Possible	Yes	No	Points Earned	Comments
1. Wears required laboratory uniform	5				
2. Walks in the laboratory area	5				
3. Reports injuries, accidents, and unsafe situations	5				
4. Keeps area clean and replaces supplies	5				
5. Washes hands frequently as needed	5				
6. Dries hands before handling electrical equipment	5				
7. Wears safety glasses	5				
8. Avoids horseplay	5				
9. Flushes solutions out of eyes or off of skin	5				
10. Informs instructor if particle gets in eye	5				
11. Operates equipment only after taught	5				
12. Reads instructions accompanying equipment	5				
13. Reports damaged or malfunctioning equipment	5				
14. Reads Material Safety Data Sheets (MSDSs) provided with hazardous chemicals	5				
15. Reads labels on solution bottles 3 times	5				
16. Handles solutions carefully to avoid contact with skin and eyes	5				
17. Reports broken equipment or spilled solutions	5				
18. Identifies patients in two (2) ways	5				
19. Explains procedures to patients	5				
20. Observes patients closely during any procedure	5				
Totals	100				

10:3 OBSERVING FIRE SAFETY

ASSIGNMENT SHEET

Grade _____ Name _____

INTRODUCTION: Knowing how to respond to a fire can save your life. This sheet will help you review the main facts of fire safety.

INSTRUCTIONS: Read the information on Observing Fire Safety. In the space provided, print the word(s) that best completes the statement or answers the question.

1. Fires need three (3) things to start. What are they?

2. List two (2) causes of fires.

3. List two (2) rules for preventing fires.

4. Where is the nearest fire alarm box located?

5. a. What is the location of the nearest fire extinguisher?

   b. What class of fire extinguisher is it? What kind of fire will it extinguish?

6. Fill in the following chart about fire extinguishers.

Class	Contains	Used on what type of fires?
A		
B		
C		
ABC		

7. For what does the acronym *RACE* stand?

   R:

   A:

   C:

   E:

8. List two (2) special precautions that must be observed when a patient is receiving oxygen.

9. Identify two (2) basic principles that must be followed when any type of disaster occurs.

10. Health care workers are _____ responsible for familiarizing themselves with disaster policies so appropriate action can be taken when a disaster strikes.

PROCEDURE 10:3 OBSERVING FIRE SAFETY

Equipment and Supplies
Fire alarm box, fire extinguishers

Procedure

1. Read the information on Observing Fire Safety.
2. Learn the four classes of fire extinguishers and know for what kind of fire each type is used.
3. Locate the nearest fire alarm box. Read the instructions on how to operate the alarm. Be sure you could set off the alarm in case of a fire.
4. Locate any fire extinguishers in the classroom or laboratory area. Look for extinguishers in both the room and surrounding building. Identify each extinguisher and the kind of fire for which it is meant to be used.
5. Learn how to operate a fire extinguisher. Read the manufacturer's operating instructions carefully. Work with a practice extinguisher or do a mock demonstration.
   CAUTION: Do *not* discharge a real extinguisher in the laboratory.

   a. Check the extinguisher type to be sure it is the proper one to use for the mock fire.
   b. Locate the lock or pin at the top handle. Following the manufacturer's instructions, release the lock and grasp the handle.
      NOTE: During a mock demonstration, only pretend to release the lock.
   c. Hold the extinguisher firmly in an upright position.
   d. Stand approximately 6 to 10 feet from the near edge of the fire.
   e. Aim the nozzle at the fire.
   f. Discharge the extinguisher. Use a side-to-side motion. Spray toward the near edge of the fire at the bottom of the fire.
      CAUTION: Do not spray into the center or top of the fire, because doing so will cause the fire to spread in an outward direction.
   g. Continue with the same motion until the fire is extinguished.
      NOTE: The word *PASS* can help you remember the correct steps:
      P = Pull the pin.
      A = Aim the extinguisher at the near edge and bottom of the fire.
      S = Squeeze the handle to discharge the extinguisher.
      S = Sweep the extinguisher from side to side.
   h. At all times, stay a safe distance from the fire to avoid personal injury.
      CAUTION: Avoid contact with residues from chemical extinguishers.
   i. After an extinguisher has been used, it must be recharged or replaced. Another usable extinguisher must be put in position when the extinguisher is removed.
6. Check the policy in your area for evacuating the laboratory area during a fire. Practice the method and know the locations of all exits.
   NOTE: Remember to remain calm and avoid panic.
7. Replace all equipment used.

Practice *Use the evaluation sheet for 10:3, Observing Fire Safety, to practice this procedure. When you feel you have mastered this skill, sign the sheet and give it to your instructor for further action.*

✔ **Final Checkpoint** Using the criteria listed on the evaluation sheet, your instructor will grade your performance.

Practice *Study the safety regulations throughout Chapter 10 in preparation for the safety examination.*

✔ **Final Checkpoint** Take the safety examination and obtain a passing grade to demonstrate your knowledge of safety.

10:3 EVALUATION SHEET

Name _____ Date _____

Evaluated by _____

DIRECTIONS: Practice fire safety according to the criteria listed. When you are ready for your final check, give this sheet to your instructor.

Observing Fire Safety	Points Possible	Yes	No	Points Earned	Comments
1. Identifies nearest alarm box	9				
2. Sounds alarm correctly	9				
3. Points out locations of extinguishers in area	9				
4. Selects correct extinguisher for following types of fires:					
Burning paper	5				
Burning oil	5				
Electrical fire	5				
5. Simulates the operation of an extinguisher:					
Checks type	5				
Releases lock	5				
Holds firmly	5				
Stands 6 to 10 feet away from edge	5				
Aims at fire	5				
Discharges correctly	5				
Uses side-to-side motion	5				
Sprays at near edge at bottom of fire	5				
6. Replaces or has extinguisher recharged after use	9				
7. Evacuates laboratory or clinical area following established policy for fires	9				
Totals	100				

CHAPTER 10 SAFETY EXAMINATION

ASSIGNMENT SHEET

Grade _____   Name _____

INSTRUCTIONS: Read all directions carefully. Put your name on all pages of the examination.

A. Multiple Choice: In the space provided, place the letter of the answer that best completes the statement or answers the question.

_____ 1. Operate a piece of equipment only when
   a. you have been instructed on how to use it
   b. you see other students using it
   c. you think you know how to handle it
   d. you have similar equipment in other classes

_____ 2. If you find a damaged piece of equipment
   a. dispose of it immediately
   b. report it to the instructor
   c. use it but be very careful
   d. repair it yourself before you use it

_____ 3. Solutions that will be used in the laboratory
   a. can be injurious, so avoid eye and skin contact
   b. can be mixed together in most cases
   c. do not always need a label
   d. are all safe for your use

_____ 4. When the instructor is out of the room
   a. equipment should not be operated
   b. it is all right to operate equipment
   c. it is a good time to experiment with equipment
   d. be extra careful when using equipment

_____ 5. All injuries that occur in the laboratory
   a. should be treated by a fellow student
   b. can be ignored if minor
   c. should be washed with soap and water
   d. should be reported to the instructor

_____ 6. If a particle gets in your eye, you should
   a. rub your eye
   b. use cotton to remove it
   c. call the instructor
   d. flush your eye with water to remove it

_____ 7. When handling any electrical equipment, be sure to
    a. wash your hands immediately before handling it
    b. check first for damaged cords or improper grounds
    c. plug equipment carefully into any socket
    d. ask for written instructions on how to use it

_____ 8. Horseplay or practical jokes
    a. are permitted if no one is insulted
    b. may be done during breaks or study time
    c. cause accidents and have no place in the lab
    d. usually do not result in accidents

_____ 9. The major cause of fires is
    a. smoking and matches
    b. defects in heating systems
    c. improper rubbish disposal
    d. misuse of electricity

_____ 10. The three things needed to start a fire are
    a. air, oxygen, and fuel
    b. fuel, heat, and oxygen
    c. fuel, carbon dioxide, and heat
    d. air, carbon dioxide, and fuel

_____ 11. Injuries are more likely to happen to persons who
    a. take chances
    b. use equipment properly
    c. practice safety
    d. respect the dangers in using equipment

_____ 12. If your personal safety is in danger because of fire
    a. get the fire extinguisher and put it out
    b. run out of the area as fast as you can
    c. leave the area quietly and in an orderly fashion
    d. open all windows and doors

_____ 13. Wearing safety glasses in a laboratory
    a. is never necessary
    b. should be done if you think it is necessary
    c. is a requirement at all times
    d. is required for certain procedures

B. True–False: Circle the T if the statement is true. Circle the F if the statement is false.

T F   1. Carbon dioxide fire extinguishers leave a residue or snow that can cause burns or eye irritations.

T F   2. Spilled solutions, such as bleach, should be wiped up immediately.

T F   3. Laboratory uniforms are worn for protection and as a safety measure.

T F   4. If any solution comes in contact with your skin or eyes, flush the area with water and call the instructor.

T F   5. The third prong on an electric plug is important for grounding electrical equipment.

T F 6. In case of a fire alarm, avoid panic.

T F 7. Correct body mechanics should be used while performing procedures.

T F 8. Class A fire extinguishers can be used on electrical fires.

T F 9. While using a fire extinguisher, hold the extinguisher firmly and direct it to the middle or main part of the fire.

T F 10. Smoke and panic kill more people in fires than the fire itself.

T F 11. For your own safety and the safety of a patient, it is important that you wash your hands frequently.

T F 12. All waste material should be disposed of in the nearest available container.

T F 13. All solutions used in the laboratory are poisonous.

T F 14. You should read the bottle label of any solution that you use at least three (3) times.

T F 15. All manufacturers must provide a Material Safety Data Sheet (MSDS) with any hazardous product they sell.

T F 16. When lifting a patient in bed, a narrow base of support should be maintained.

T F 17. Keep the feet apart and the knees flexed when picking up an item from the floor.

C. Completion or Short Answer: In the space provided, print the word(s) that best completes the statement or answers the question.

1. Fill in the following chart with the indicated information.

Type Fire Extinguisher	Contains	Used on what type of fire?

a. _____

b. _____

c. _____

d. _____

2. List two (2) rules for preventing fires.

3. What is OSHA? What is its purpose?

4. How can you determine precautions that should be followed while using a hazardous chemical?

5. Identify two (2) diseases that can be contracted by exposure to body fluids.

CHAPTER 10 INTERNET SEARCHES

Use the suggested search engines in Chapter 9:4 of the textbook to search the Internet for additional information on the following topics:

1. *Federal regulations:* Obtain more information on federal safety regulations by searching sites of the Occupational Safety and Health Administration (OSHA), Occupational Exposure to Hazardous Chemicals Standard, Bloodborne Pathogen Standard, and Material Safety Data Sheets (MSDS).

2. *Ergonomics:* Search for additional information on ergonomics and environmental safety.

3. *Diseases:* Obtain information on hepatitis B and C and acquired immune deficiency syndrome (AIDS). Learn the cause of the diseases and how to prevent them from spreading.

4. *Fire safety:* Search for information on fire prevention and fire safety.

5. *Fire extinguishers:* Search for various manufacturers of fire extinguishers. Obtain information on the types of extinguishers, their main uses, precautions for handling, and safety rules that must be observed while using extinguishers.

6. *Disasters:* Obtain information on safety procedures that must be followed for tornadoes, floods, hurricanes, and earthquakes.

11:1 UNDERSTANDING THE PRINCIPLES OF INFECTION CONTROL

ASSIGNMENT SHEET

Grade _____   Name _____

INTRODUCTION: This assignment will allow you to gain a basic knowledge of how disease is transmitted and the main ways to prevent it.

INSTRUCTIONS: Read the information on Understanding the Principles of Infection Control. In the space provided, print the word(s) that best completes the statement or answers the question.

1. Use the Key Terms to complete the crossword puzzle.

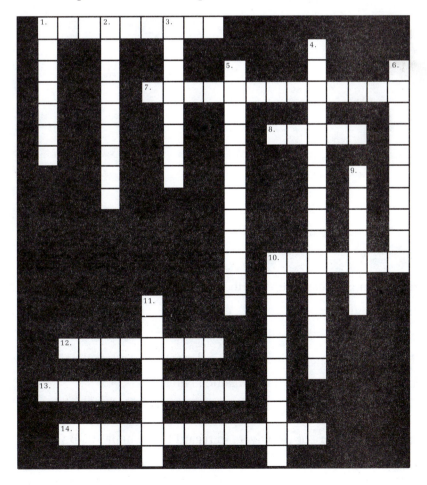

ACROSS

1. Organisms that live and reproduce in the absence of oxygen

7. Process that destroys all microorganisms including spores and viruses

8. Plantlike organisms that live on dead organic matter

10. Absence of pathogens

12. Germ- or disease-producing microorganism

13. Infections acquired in a health care facility

14. Small living plant or animal organism not visible to naked eye

DOWN

1. Organisms that require oxygen to live

2. Disease originates outside the body

3. One-celled plantlike organisms that multiply rapidly

4. Factors that must be present for disease to occur

5. Process that destroys or kills pathogens

6. Disease originates within the body

9. Smallest microorganisms

10. Process that inhibits or prevents the growth of pathogenic organisms

11. One-celled animal organisms found in decayed materials and contaminated water

2. How do nonpathogens differ from pathogens?

3. Identify the following shapes of bacteria.

   a. rod shaped:

   b. comma shaped:

   c. round or spherical arranged in a chain:

   d. spiral or corkscrew:

4. Identify the class of microorganisms described by the following statements.

   a. smallest microorganisms:

   b. parasitic microorganisms:

   c. one-celled animal organisms found in decayed materials and contaminated water:

   d. plantlike organisms that live on dead organic matter:

   e. microorganisms that live on fleas, lice, ticks, and mites:

5. What does federal law require of employers in regard to the hepatitis B vaccine?

6. List three (3) things needed for microorganisms to grow and reproduce.

7. What is the difference between an endogenous disease and an exogenous disease?

8. Name two (2) common examples of nosocomial infections.

9. What do health care facilities do to prevent and deal with nosocomial infections?

10. Identify the part(s) of the chain of infection that has been eliminated by the following actions.

    a. thorough washing of the hands:

    b. intact, unbroken skin:

    c. healthy, well-rested individual:

    d. cleaning and sterilizing a blood-covered instrument:

    e. spraying to destroy mosquitoes:

11. List three (3) common aseptic techniques.

12. Define the following.

    a. antisepsis:

    b. disinfection:

    c. sterilization:

11:2 WASHING HANDS

ASSIGNMENT SHEET

Grade _____ Name _____

INTRODUCTION: Handwashing is the most important method used to practice aseptic technique. This assignment will help you review the main facts.

INSTRUCTIONS: Read the information on Washing Hands. In the space provided, print the word(s) that best completes the statement or answers the question.

1. List two (2) reasons for washing the hands.

2. List five (5) times the hands should be washed.

3. Why is soap used as a cleansing agent?

4. How should the fingertips be pointed while washing hands?

   Why?

5. What temperature water should be used?

   Why?

6. Why are paper towels used while turning on and off the faucet?

7. List three (3) surfaces on the hands that must be cleaned.

8. Name two (2) items that can be used to clean the nails.

Equipment and Supplies

Paper towels, running water, waste container, hand brush or orange/cuticle stick, soap

Procedure

1. Assemble all equipment. Stand back slightly from the sink so you do not contaminate your uniform or clothing. Avoid touching the inside of the sink with your hands because it is considered contaminated.

2. Turn on the faucet by holding a paper towel between your hand and the faucet. Regulate the temperature of the water until it is warm. Let the water flow over your hands. Discard the towel in the waste container.

   NOTE: Water should be warm.

   CAUTION: Hot water will burn your hands.

3. With your fingertips pointing downward, wet your hands.

   NOTE: Washing in a downward direction prevents water from getting on the forearms and then running back down to contaminate hands.

4. Use soap to get a lather on your hands.

5. Put the palms of your hands together and rub them using friction and a circular motion for approximately 10 to 15 seconds.

6. Put the palm of one hand on the back of the other hand. Rub together several times. Repeat this after reversing position of hands.

7. Interlace the fingers on both hands and rub them back and forth.

8. Clean the nails with an orange/cuticle stick and/or hand brush.

   CAUTION: Use the blunt end of the orange/cuticle stick to avoid injury.

   NOTE: Steps 3 through 8 ensure that all parts of both hands are clean.

9. Rinse your hands, keeping fingertips pointed downward.

10. Use a clean paper towel to dry hands thoroughly, from tips of fingers to wrist. Discard the towel in the waste container.

11. Use another dry paper towel to turn off the faucet.

    CAUTION: Wet towels allow passage of pathogens.

12. Discard all used towels in the waste container. Leave the area neat and clean.

Practice *Use the evaluation sheet for 11:2, Washing Hands, to practice this procedure. When you feel you have mastered this skill, sign the sheet and give it to your instructor for further action.*

✔ **Final Checkpoint** Using the criteria listed on the evaluation sheet, your instructor will grade your performance.

11:2 EVALUATION SHEET

Name _____ Date _____

Evaluated by _____

DIRECTIONS: Practice washing hands according to the criteria listed. When you are ready for your final check, give this sheet to your instructor.

Washing Hands	Points Possible	Yes	No	Points Earned	Comments
1. Assembles supplies	5				
2. Turns on faucet using dry towel	6				
3. Regulates temperature of water	6				
4. Wets hands with fingertips pointed down	7				
5. Gets soapy lather	6				
6. Scrubs palms using friction and a circular motion for 10 to 15 seconds	7				
7. Scrubs tops of hands with opposite palms	7				
8. Interlaces fingers to wash between	7				
9. Cleans nails:					
With small brush	5				
Uses blunt edge of orange stick	5				
10. Rinses with fingertips pointed down	7				
11. Dries thoroughly	7				
12. Places towels in waste can	6				
13. Turns off faucet using dry towel	7				
14. Leaves area neat and clean	5				
15. Identifies three (3) times hands must be washed	7				
Totals	100				

11:3 OBSERVING STANDARD PRECAUTIONS

ASSIGNMENT SHEET

Grade _____ Name _____

INTRODUCTION: Observing standard precautions is one way the chain of infection can be broken. This assignment will allow you to review the main principles of standard precautions.

INSTRUCTIONS: Read the information on Observing Standard Precautions. In the space provided, print the word(s) that best completes the statement or answers the question.

1. Name three (3) pathogens spread by blood and body fluids that are a major concern to health care workers.

2. What federal agency established standards for preventing contamination with blood or body fluids that must be followed by all health care facilities?

3. Name three (3) types of personal protective equipment (PPE) that an employer must provide.

4. Can a health care worker drink coffee in a laboratory where blood tests are performed? Why or why not?

5. What responsibilities does an employer have if an employee is splashed with blood when a tube containing blood breaks?

6. List the three (3) requirements that employers must meet as a result of the Needlestick Safety and Prevention Act.

7. When must standard precautions be used?

8. Describe three (3) situations when gloves must be worn.

9. When must gowns be worn?

10. Describe two (2) examples of situations when masks, protective eyewear, or face shields must be worn.

11. When must masks be changed?

12. How must needles and syringes be handled after use?

13. During a blood test, some blood splashes on the laboratory counter. How must it be removed?

14. What is the purpose of mouthpieces or resuscitation devices?

15. What must you do if you stick yourself with a contaminated needle?

PROCEDURE 11:3 OBSERVING STANDARD PRECAUTIONS

Equipment and Supplies

Disposable gloves, infectious waste bags, needle and syringe, sharps container, gown, masks, protective eyewear, resuscitation devices

NOTE: This procedure will help you learn standard precautions. It is important for you to observe these precautions at all times while working in the laboratory or clinical area.

Procedure

1. Assemble equipment.

2. Review the precautions in the textbook for Observing Standard Precautions. Note points that are not clear, and ask your instructor for an explanation.

3. Practice handwashing according to Procedure 11:2. Identify at least five times that hands must be washed according to standard precautions.

4. Name three instances when gloves must be worn to observe standard precautions. Put on a pair of disposable gloves. Practice removing the gloves without contaminating the skin. With a gloved hand, grasp the cuff of the glove on the opposite hand, handling only the outside of the glove. Pull the glove down and turn it inside out while removing it. Take care not to touch the skin with the gloved hand. Using the ungloved hand, slip the fingers under the cuff of the glove on the opposite hand. Touching only the inside of the glove and taking care not to touch the skin, pull the glove down and turn it inside out while removing it. Place the gloves in an infectious waste container. Wash your hands immediately.

5. Practice putting on a gown. State when a gown is to be worn. To remove the gown, touch only the inside. Fold the contaminated gown so the outside is folded inward. Roll it into a bundle and place it in an infectious waste container if it is disposable. Place it in a bag for contaminated linen if it is not disposable.

   CAUTION: If a gown is contaminated, gloves should be worn while removing the gown.

   NOTE: Folding the gown and rolling it prevents transmission of pathogens.

6. Practice putting on a mask and protective eyewear. To remove the mask, handle it by the ties only. Clean and disinfect protective eyewear after use.

7. Practice proper disposal of sharps. Uncap a needle attached to a syringe, taking care not to stick yourself with the needle. Place the entire needle and syringe in a sharps container. State the rules regarding disposal of the sharps container.

8. Spill a small amount of water on a counter. Pretend that it is blood. Put on gloves and use disposable cloths or gauze to wipe up the spill. Put the contaminated cloths or gauze in an infectious waste bag. Use clean disposable cloths or gauze to wipe the area thoroughly with a disinfectant agent. Put the cloths or gauze in the infectious waste bag, remove your gloves, and wash your hands.

9. Practice handling an infectious waste bag. Fold down the top edge of the bag to form a cuff at the top of the bag. Wear gloves to close the bag after contaminated wastes have been placed in it. Put your hands under the folded cuff and gently expel excess air from the bag. Twist the top of the bag shut and fold down the top edges to seal the bag. Secure the fold with tape or a tie according to agency policy.

10. Examine mouthpieces and resuscitation devices that can be used in place of mouth-to-mouth resuscitation. You will be taught to use these devices when you learn cardiopulmonary resuscitation (CPR).

11. Discuss the following situations with another student and determine which standard precautions should be observed:

    ■ A patient has an open sore on the skin, and pus is seeping from the area. You are going to bathe the patient.

Procedure 11:3 (cont.)

- You are cleaning a tray of instruments that contains a disposable surgical blade and needle with syringe.
- A tube of blood drops to the floor and breaks, spilling the blood on the floor.
- Drainage from dressings on an infected wound has soiled the linen on the bed you are changing.
- You work in a dental office and are assisting a dentist while a tooth is being extracted (removed).

12. Replace all equipment used.

Practice *Use the evaluation sheet for 11:3, Observing Standard Precautions. When you feel you have mastered this skill, sign the sheet and give it to your instructor for further action.*

✔ **Final Checkpoint** Using the criteria listed on the evaluation sheet, your instructor will grade your performance.

11:3 EVALUATION SHEET

Name _____ Date _____

Evaluated by _____

DIRECTIONS: Practice observing standard precautions according to the criteria listed. When you are ready for your final check, give this sheet to your instructor.

Observing Standard Precautions	Points Possible	Yes	No	Points Earned	Comments
1. Assembles equipment and supplies	3				
2. Washes hands correctly	4				
3. Puts on gloves if:					
Contacting blood, body fluid, secretions, excretions, mucous membranes, or nonintact skin	3				
Handling contaminated items/surfaces	3				
Performing invasive procedures	3				
Performing blood tests	3				
4. Removes gloves correctly:					
Grasps outside of cuff of first glove	3				
Pulls glove down and turns inside out	3				
Places fingers inside cuff of second glove	4				
Pulls glove down and turns inside out	3				
Disposes of gloves correctly	3				
Washes hands immediately	3				
5. Puts on gown if splashing of blood/body fluid likely	4				
6. Removes gown correctly:					
Handles only inside while removing	2				
Folds gown inward	2				
Rolls gown	2				
Places in proper laundry bag	2				
7. Wears masks and protective eyewear if needed:					
Puts on if droplets of blood/body fluid likely	3				
Handles only ties of mask when removing	3				
Cleans and disinfects protective eyewear	3				
8. Disposes of sharps correctly	4				

Observing Standard Precautions	Points Possible	Yes	No	Points Earned	Comments
9. Wipes up spills/splashes of blood/body fluids:					
Puts on gloves	2				
Wipes up spill with disposable cloths/gauze	2				
Discards cloths/gauze in infectious waste bag	2				
Wipes area with clean cloth/gauze and disinfectant	2				
Discards cloths/gauze in infectious waste bag	2				
Removes gloves	2				
Washes hands immediately	2				
10. Handles infectious waste bags correctly:					
Forms cuff at top before using	2				
Discards infectious waste in bag	2				
Wears gloves to close bag	2				
Puts hands under cuff	2				
Expels excess air gently	2				
Folds top edges to seal bag	2				
Tapes or ties bag	2				
11. Uses mouthpieces or resuscitation devices correctly	4				
12. Replaces equipment	2				
13. Washes hands	3				
Totals	100				

11:4 MAINTAINING TRANSMISSION-BASED ISOLATION PRECAUTIONS

ASSIGNMENT SHEET

Grade _____ Name _____

INTRODUCTION: Transmission-based isolation techniques will vary from area to area, but the same principles are observed in all types. This sheet will help you review these main principles.

INSTRUCTIONS: Read the text information on Maintaining Transmission-Based Isolation Precautions. In the space provided, print the word(s) that best completes the statement or answers the question.

1. Define *transmission-based isolation*.

2. What is the difference between standard precautions and transmission-based isolation techniques?

3. What is a communicable disease?

4. List two (2) ways communicable diseases are spread.

5. Identify two (2) factors that help determine what type of isolation is used.

6. Define *contaminated*.

7. Define *clean*.

8. Using the guidelines established by the Centers for Disease Control and Prevention (CDC), place the letter or letters for the type of isolation used in Column B by any statement in Column A that pertains to this type of isolation.

Column A

     1. Used for measles and tuberculosis

     2. Used for all patients

     3. Gloves must be worn when entering room

     4. Used for wound infections caused by multidrug-resistant organisms

     5. Anyone entering room must wear high-efficiency particulate air (HEPA) mask

     6. Masks must be worn when working within 3 feet of patient

     7. Room and items in it should receive daily cleaning and disinfection

     8. Patient should be placed in a private room

     9. Used for pathogens transmitted by large particle droplets

    10. Room air should be discharged to outdoor air or filtered

Column B

A. Airborne

B. Contact

C. Droplet

D. Standard

9. What is protective or reverse isolation?

10. List two (2) types of patients who may require protective or reverse isolation.

NOTE: The following procedure deals with contact transmission-based isolation precautions. For other types of transmission-based isolation, follow only the steps that apply.

Equipment and Supplies

Isolation gown, surgical mask, gloves, small plastic bag, linen cart or container, infectious waste container, paper towels, sink with running water

Procedure

1. Assemble equipment.

   NOTE: In many agencies, clean isolation garments and supplies are kept on a cart outside the isolation unit or in the outer room of a two-room unit. A waste container should be positioned just inside the door.

2. Wash hands.

3. Remove rings and place them in your pocket or pin them to your uniform.

4. Remove your watch and place it in a small plastic bag or centered on a clean paper towel. If placed on a towel, handle only the bottom part of the towel; do not touch the top.

   NOTE: The watch will be taken into the room and placed on the bedside stand for taking vital signs. Because it cannot be sterilized, it must be kept clean.

   NOTE: In some agencies, a plastic-covered watch is left in the isolation room.

5. Put on the mask. Secure it under your chin. Make sure to cover your mouth and nose. Handle the mask as little as possible. Tie the mask securely behind your head and neck. Tie the top ties first and the bottom ties second.

   NOTE: The tie bands on the mask are considered clean. The mask is considered contaminated.

   NOTE: The mask is considered to be contaminated after 30 minutes in isolation or anytime it gets wet. If you remain in isolation longer than 30 minutes, or if the mask gets wet, you must wash your hands and remove and discard the old mask. Then wash your hands again and put on a clean mask.

6. If uniform sleeves are long, roll them up above the elbows before putting on the gown.

7. Lift the gown by placing your hands inside the shoulders.

   NOTE: The inside of the gown and the ties at the neck are considered clean.

   NOTE: Most agencies use disposable gowns that are discarded after use.

8. Work your arms into the sleeves of the gown by gentle twisting. Take care not to touch your face with the sleeves of the gown.

9. Place your hands *inside* the neckband, adjust until it is in position, and then tie the bands at the back of your neck.

10. Reach behind and fold the edges of the gown over so that the uniform is completely covered. Tie the waistbands. Some waistbands are long enough to wrap around your body before tying.

11. If gloves are to be worn, put them on. Make sure that the cuff of the glove comes over the top of the cuff of the gown. In this way, there are no open areas for entrance of organisms.

12. You are now ready to enter the isolation room. Double check to be sure you have all equipment and supplies that you will need for patient care before you enter the room.

13. When patient care is complete, you will be ready to remove isolation garments. In a two-room isolation unit, go to the outer room. In a one-room unit, remove garments while you are standing close to the inside of the door. Take care to avoid touching the room's contaminated articles.

Procedure 11:4 (cont.)

14. Untie the waist ties. Loosen the gown at the waist.

    NOTE: The waist ties are considered contaminated.

15. If gloves are worn, remove the first glove by grasping the outside of the cuff with the opposite gloved hand. Pull the glove over the hand so that the glove is inside out. Remove the second glove by placing the bare hand inside the cuff. Pull the glove off so it is inside out. Place the disposable gloves in the infectious waste container.

16. To avoid unnecessary transmission of organisms, use paper towels to turn on the water faucet. Wash and dry your hands thoroughly. When they are dry, use a clean, dry paper towel to turn off the faucet.

    CAUTION: Organisms travel rapidly through wet towels.

17. Untie the mask. Holding the mask by the ties only, drop it into the infectious waste container.

    NOTE: The ties of the mask are considered clean. Do not touch any other part of the mask because it is considered contaminated.

18. Untie the neck ties. Loosen the gown at the shoulders, handling only the inside of the gown.

    NOTE: The neck ties are considered clean.

19. Slip the fingers of one hand inside the opposite cuff. Do *not* touch the outside. Pull the sleeve down over the hand.

    CAUTION: The outside of the gown is considered contaminated and should not be touched.

20. Using the gown-covered hand, pull the sleeve down over the opposite hand.

21. Ease your arms and hands out of the gown. Keep the gown in front of your body and keep your hands away from the outside of the gown. Use as gentle a motion as possible.

    NOTE: Excessive flapping of the gown will spread organisms.

22. With your hands inside the gown at the shoulders, bring the shoulders together and turn the gown so that it is inside out. In this manner, the outside of the contaminated gown is on the inside. Fold the gown in half and then roll it together. Place it in the infectious waste container.

    NOTE: Avoid excess motion during this procedure because motion causes the spread of organisms.

23. Wash hands thoroughly. Use dry, clean paper towels to operate the faucets.

24. Touch only the inside of the plastic bag to remove your watch. Discard the bag in the waste container. If the watch is on a paper towel, handle only the "clean," top portion (if necessary). Discard the towel in the infectious waste container.

25. Use a clean paper towel to open the door. Discard the towel in the waste container before leaving the room.

    CAUTION: The inside of the door is considered contaminated.

    NOTE: The waste container should be positioned just inside the door of the room.

26. After leaving the isolation room, wash hands thoroughly. This will help prevent spread of the disease. It also protects you from the illness.

Practice *Use the evaluation sheet for 11:4, Donning and Removing Transmission-Based Isolation Garments, to practice this procedure. When you feel you have mastered this skill, sign the sheet and give it to your instructor for further action.*

✔ **Final Checkpoint** Using the criteria listed on the evaluation sheet, your instructor will grade your performance.

11:4 EVALUATION SHEET

Name _____ Date _____

Evaluated by _____

DIRECTIONS: Practice donning and removing transmission-based isolation garments according to the criteria listed. When you are ready for your final check, give this sheet to your instructor.

Donning and Removing Transmission-Based Isolation Garments	Points Possible	Yes	No	Points Earned	Comments
1. Assembles equipment and supplies	4				
2. Washes hands	4				
3. Removes rings	4				
4. Places watch in plastic bag or on paper towel	4				
5. Applies mask correctly:					
Handles very little	2				
Covers mouth and nose	2				
Ties in back securely	2				
Changes mask every 30 minutes or anytime it gets wet	2				
6. Rolls up uniform sleeves	3				
7. Puts on gown correctly:					
Keeps hands inside shoulders	2				
Works arms in gently	2				
Adjusts neck with hands inside neck band	2				
Ties at neck first	2				
Ties at waist	2				
Handles only inside of gown	3				
8. Applies gloves correctly:	3				
Covers cuffs of gown with gloves	3				
Removal of Garments:					
9. Unties waist ties of gown first	3				
10. Removes gloves:					
Uses gloves hand to grasp outside of opposite glove	2				
Pulls glove off inside out	2				
Places ungloved hand under cuff to remove second glove	2				
Pulls glove off inside out	2				
Places gloves in infectious waste container	2				

161

Donning and Removing Transmission-Based Isolation Garments	Points Possible	Yes	No	Points Earned	Comments
11. Washes hands thoroughly:	3				
Uses towel to operate faucet	3				
12. Removes mask after gloves:	2				
Handles ties only	2				
Places in infectious waste container	2				
13. Removes gown last:	2				
Unties neck ties	2				
Places one hand inside cuff and pulls sleeve over hand	2				
Places covered hand on outside of gown to pull gown sleeve over second hand	2				
Eases out of gown gently	2				
Folds gown so inside of gown is on outside	2				
Rolls gown	2				
Places gown in linen hamper (or infectious-waste can if gown disposable)	2				
Touches only inside of gown	3				
14. Washes hands thoroughly	3				
15. Removes watch by touching only inside of plastic bag or top part of towel	2				
16. Opens door with towel, discards towel in waste can	2				
17. Washes hands immediately	3				
Totals	100				

11:5 BIOTERRORISM

ASSIGNMENT SHEET

Grade _____ Name _____

INTRODUCTION: This assignment will allow you to gain a basic knowledge about bioterrorism and how to prevent it.

INSTRUCTIONS: Read the information on Bioterrorism. In the space provided, print the word(s) that best completes the statement or answers the question.

1. Define *bioterrorism*.

2. List two (2) examples of how bioterrorism was used during wars.

3. Identify four (4) characteristics of an "ideal" microorganism for bioterrorism.

4. Name the following high-priority bioterrorism agents identified by the CDC.
   a. highly contagious disease caused by a variola virus that can be prevented with a vaccine:

   b. a bacterium commonly found in animals such as rats, rabbits, and insects that can be treated with antibiotics:

   c. organisms that cause severe hemorrhagic fever:

   d. a bacterium that produces a toxin causing paralysis of muscles:

   e. an infectious disease caused by spores that can live in the soil for years:

5. What is the name of the law passed by Congress in 2002 to deal with bioterrorism?

6. List five (5) things that can be done to prepare for a bioterrorism attack.

CHAPTER 11 INTERNET SEARCHES

Use the suggested search engines in Chapter 9:4 of the textbook to search the Internet for additional information on the following topics:

1. *Organizations regulating infection control:* Find the organization sites for the Occupational Safety and Health Administration (OSHA), Centers for Disease Control and Prevention (CDC), National Center for Infectious Diseases (NCID), and the Hospital Infection Control Practices Advisory Committee (HICPAC) to obtain information on regulations governing infection control.

2. *Microbiology:* Search for specific information on bacteria (can also search for specific types such as *Escherichia coli*), protozoa, fungi, rickettsiae, and viruses.

3. *Diseases:* Obtain information on the method of transmission, signs and symptoms, treatment, and complications for diseases such as hepatitis B, hepatitis C, acquired immune deficiency syndrome, and specific diseases listed by the discussion on microorganisms in this chapter.

4. *Infections:* Research endogenous infections, exogenous infections, nosocomial infections, and opportunistic infections.

5. *Infection control:* Locate and read the Bloodborne Pathogen Standards, Needlestick Safety and Prevention Act, Standard Precautions, and Transmission-Based Isolation Precautions (airborne precautions, droplet precautions, and contact precautions).

6. *Medical supply companies:* Search for names of specific medical supply companies to research products available such as autoclaves, chemical disinfectants, and spill clean-up kits.

CHAPTER 12 VITAL SIGNS

12:1 MEASURING AND RECORDING VITAL SIGNS

ASSIGNMENT SHEET

Grade _____ Name _____

INTRODUCTION: Vital signs are important indicators of health states of the body. This assignment will help you review the main facts about vital signs.

INSTRUCTIONS: Read the information on Measuring and Recording Vital Signs. In the space provided, print the word(s) that best completes the statements or answers the questions.

1. Use the Key Terms to complete the crossword puzzle.

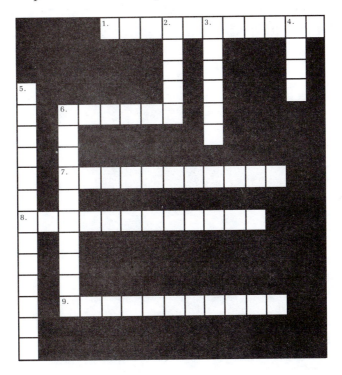

ACROSS

1. Measurement of the balance between heat lost and heat produced

6. Strength of the pulse

7. Pulse taken at the apex of the heart with a stethoscope

8. Measurement of breaths taken by a patient

9. Instrument used to take apical pulse

DOWN

2. Pressure of the blood felt against the wall of an artery

3. Regularity of the pulse or respirations

4. Number of beats per minute

5. Measurement of the force exerted by the heart against arterial walls

6. Various determinations that provide information about body conditions

2. List the four (4) main vital signs.

3. Why is it essential that vital signs be measured accurately?

4. Define *pulse*.

5. List three (3) factors recorded about a pulse.

6. What three (3) factors are noted about respirations?

7. Identify the two (2) readings noted on a blood pressure.

8. List two (2) situations where you may have to take an apical pulse.

9. What should you do if you note an abnormality or change in any vital sign?

10. What should you do if you are not able to obtain a correct reading for a vital sign?

12:2 MEASURING AND RECORDING TEMPERATURE

ASSIGNMENT SHEET

Grade _____ Name _____

INTRODUCTION: In addition to being able to take temperatures, it will be important for you to know the main facts about body temperature. This assignment will help you review these facts.

INSTRUCTIONS: Read the information on Measuring and Recording Temperature. In the space provided, print the word(s) that best completes the statements or answers the questions.

1. Define *temperature*.

2. List three main reasons why temperature may vary.

3. The normal range for body temperature is _____ to _____ degrees Fahrenheit.

4. A normal oral temperature is _____ degrees Fahrenheit. The clinical thermometer is left in place for _____ minutes.

5. A normal rectal temperature is _____ degrees Fahrenheit. The clinical thermometer is left in place for _____ minutes.

6. A normal axillary temperature is _____ degrees Fahrenheit. The clinical thermometer is left in place for _____ minutes.

7. What is the most accurate method for taking a temperature? Why?

8. What is the least accurate method for taking a temperature? Why?

9. What is an aural temperature?

   How does an aural thermometer measure temperature?

10. What is the difference between hyperthermia and hypothermia?

11. List two (2) ways you can tell a rectal clinical thermometer from an oral clinical thermometer.

12. Why do OSHA, the EPA, and the AMA all discourage the use of mercury-filled clinical thermometers?

13. How can you prevent cross-contamination while using the probe of an electronic thermometer?

14. How do plastic or paper thermometers register body temperature?

15. Why is it important to ask patients if they have had anything to eat or drink or if they have smoked before taking an oral temperature?

16. How long should a thermometer soak in a disinfectant (after cleaning) before it is safe to rinse in cold water and use on a patient?

READING A THERMOMETER

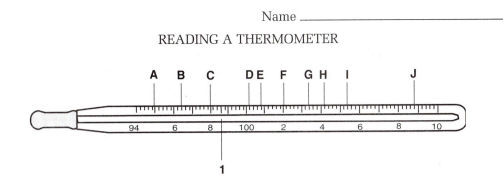

17. After the following steps is a list of temperatures that are to be recorded along the bottom of the illustrated thermometer:

■ Each temperature reading is preceded by a listed number (1, 2, 3, etc.).

■ Locate the line on the sketch that reflects the temperature reading.

■ Draw an arrow to the correct line on the thermometer.

■ Place the listed number below the arrow (1, 2, 3, etc.).

■ See Example 1.

1. 98^6 (Example)

2. 100^4

3. 99

4. 99^8

5. 102^6

6. 104^4

7. 97^6

8. 95^4

9. 101^2

10. 106^8

18. Note that in the sketch in question 17, letters appear along the top of the thermometer. Each letter has an arrow pointing to a line on the thermometer. This is the temperature reading. Record each reading beside the corresponding letter that follows. (Note Example A.)

A. 95 (Example)

B.

C.

D.

E.

F.

G.

H.

I.

J.

Equipment and Supplies

Oral thermometer, plastic sheath (if used), holder with disinfectant solution, tissues or dry cotton balls, container for used tissues, watch with second hand, soapy cotton balls, disposable gloves, notepaper, pencil/pen

Procedure

1. Assemble equipment.

2. Wash hands and put on gloves.

   CAUTION: Follow standard precautions for contact with saliva or the mucous membrane of the mouth.

3. Introduce yourself. Identify the patient. Explain the procedure.

4. Position the patient comfortably. Ask the patient whether he or she has eaten, has had hot or cold fluids, or has smoked in the past 15 minutes.

   NOTE: Eating, drinking liquids, or smoking can affect the temperature in the mouth. Wait at least 15 minutes if the patient says yes to your question.

5. Remove the clean thermometer by the upper end. Use a clean tissue or dry cotton ball to wipe the thermometer from stem to bulb.

   NOTE: If the thermometer was soaking in a disinfectant, rinse first in cool water.

   CAUTION: Hold the thermometer securely to avoid breaking.

6. Read the thermometer to be sure it reads 96°F (35.6°C) or lower. Check carefully for chips or breaks.

   CAUTION: Never use a cracked thermometer because it may injure the patient.

   NOTE: If a plastic sheath is used, place it on the thermometer after checking for damage.

7. Insert the bulb under the patient's tongue, toward the side of the mouth. Ask the patient to hold it in place with the lips. Caution against biting it.

   NOTE: Check to be sure patient's mouth is closed.

8. Leave the thermometer in place for 3 to 5 minutes.

   NOTE: Some agencies require that the thermometer be left in place for 5 to 8 minutes. Follow your agency's policy.

9. Remove the thermometer. Hold it by the stem and use a tissue or cotton ball to wipe toward the bulb.

   NOTE: If a plastic sheath was used to cover the thermometer, there is no need to wipe the thermometer. Simply remove the sheath, taking care not to touch the part that was in the patient's mouth.

   CAUTION: Do *not* hold the bulb end. Doing so could alter the reading because of the warmth of your hand.

10. Read the thermometer. Record the reading on notepaper.

    NOTE: Recheck the reading and your notation for accuracy.

    NOTE: If the reading is less than 97°F, reinsert the thermometer in the patient's mouth for 1 to 2 minutes.

11. Clean the thermometer as instructed. Shake down to 96°F (35.6°C) or lower for next use.

12. Check the patient for comfort and safety before leaving.

Procedure 12:2A (cont.)

13. Replace all equipment.

14. Remove gloves and discard in infectious waste container. Wash hands.

15. Record required information on the patient's chart or agency form, for example, date and time, T 98^6, your signature and title. Report any abnormal reading to your supervisor immediately.

Practice *Use the evaluation sheet for 12:2A, Measuring and Recording Oral Temperature with a Clinical Thermometer, to practice this procedure. When you feel you have mastered this skill, sign the sheet and give it to your instructor for further action.*

✔**Final Checkpoint** Using the criteria listed on the evaluation sheet, your instructor will grade your performance.

12:2A EVALUATION SHEET

Name _____ Date _____

Evaluated by _____

DIRECTIONS: Practice measuring and recording an oral temperature with a clinical thermometer according to the criteria listed. When you are ready for your final check, give this sheet to your instructor.

Measuring and Recording Oral Temperature with a Clinical Thermometer	Points Possible	Yes	No	Points Earned	Comments
1. Assembles equipment and supplies	4				
2. Washes hands and puts on gloves	5				
3. Introduces self and identifies patient	4				
4. Explains procedure	4				
5. Questions patient on eating, drinking, or smoking	6				
6. Wipes thermometer	4				
7. Checks and reads thermometer and applies sheath if used	6				
8. Instructs patient on holding it in mouth	6				
9. Cautions against biting thermometer	6				
10. Leaves in place 3 to 5 minutes	6				
11. Removes and wipes or removes sheath, and holds at stem end for reading	6				
12. Reads to nearest two-tenths of a degree	8				
13. Records correctly	8				
14. Cleans correctly:					
Wipes with soapy cotton ball	3				
Rinses in cool water	3				
Shakes down correctly	3				
Soaks proper time	3				
15. Replaces all equipment	4				
16. Removes gloves and washes hands	5				
17. Recognizes an abnormal reading and reports it immediately	6				
Totals	100				

Name _____

PROCEDURE 12:2B MEASURING ORAL TEMPERATURE WITH AN ELECTRONIC THERMOMETER

Equipment and Supplies

Electronic thermometer with probe, sheath (probe cover), paper, pen/pencil, container for soiled sheath

Procedure

1. Assemble equipment.

   NOTE: Read the operating instructions for the electronic thermometer so you understand how the particular model operates.

2. Wash hands. Put on gloves.

   CAUTION: Follow standard precautions and wear gloves if you are taking an oral temperature.

3. Introduce yourself. Identify the patient. Explain the procedure.

4. Position the patient comfortably. Ask the patient if he or she has eaten, has had hot or cold fluids, or has smoked in the past 15 minutes. Wait at least 15 minutes if the patient answers yes.

5. If the probe has to be connected to the thermometer unit, insert the probe into the correct receptacle. If the thermometer has an "on" or "activate" button, push the button to turn on the thermometer.

6. Cover the probe with the sheath or probe cover.

7. Insert the covered probe under the patient's tongue, toward the side of the mouth. Ask the patient to close his or her lips over the probe. Caution the patient not to bite down on the probe. Most probes are heavy, so it is usually necessary to hold the probe in position.

8. When the unit signals that the temperature has been recorded, remove the probe.

   NOTE: Many electronic thermometers have an audible "beep." Others indicate that temperature has been recorded when the numbers stop flashing and become stationary.

9. Read and record the temperature. Recheck your reading for accuracy.

10. Without touching the sheath or probe cover, remove it from the probe. Many thermometers have a button you push to remove the sheath. Discard the sheath in an infectious waste container.

11. Reposition the patient. Observe all safety checkpoints before leaving the patient.

12. Return the probe to the correct storage position in the thermometer unit. Turn off the unit if necessary. Place the unit in the charging stand if the model has a charging unit.

13. Replace all equipment.

14. Remove gloves and discard in an infectious waste container. Wash hands.

15. Record required information on the patient's chart or agency form, for example, date and time, T 98^8, your signature and title. Report any abnormal reading to your supervisor immediately.

Practice *Use the evaluation sheet for 12:2B, Measuring Oral Temperature with an Electronic Thermometer, to practice this procedure. When you feel you have mastered this skill, sign the sheet and give it to your instructor for further action.*

✔ **Final Checkpoint** Using the criteria listed on the evaluation sheet, your instructor will grade your performance.

173

12:2B EVALUATION SHEET

Name _____ Date _____

Evaluated by _____

DIRECTIONS: Practice measuring and recording oral temperature with an electrical thermometer according to the criteria listed. When you are ready for your final check, give this sheet to your instructor.

Measuring Oral Temperature with an Electronic Thermometer	Points Possible	Yes	No	Points Earned	Comments
1. Assembles equipment and supplies	4				
2. Washes hands and puts on gloves	5				
3. Introduces self and identifies patient	4				
4. Explains procedure	4				
5. Positions patient correctly and questions patient on eating, drinking, or smoking	7				
6. If necessary, inserts probe into thermometer unit and turns on unit	6				
7. Covers probe with sheath or probe cover	6				
8. Inserts probe into mouth correctly and holds probe in position	7				
9. Removes probe when thermometer signals that temperature has been recorded	7				
10. Reads thermometer correctly	8				
11. Records correctly	8				
12. Removes and discards sheath or probe cover correctly	6				
13. Repositions patient for comfort and safety	6				
14. If necessary, positions probe in correct storage position in thermometer unit and turns off unit	6				
15. Replaces all equipment	4				
16. Removes gloves and washes hands	5				
17. Recognizes an abnormal reading and reports it immediately	7				
Totals	100				

174   Copyright © 2004 by Delmar Learning, a division of Thomson Learning, Inc. ALL RIGHTS RESERVED.

PROCEDURE 12:2C MEASURING AND RECORDING TYMPANIC (AURAL) TEMPERATURE

Equipment and Supplies

Tympanic thermometer, probe cover, paper, pencil/pen, container for soiled probe cover

Procedure

1. Assemble equipment.

   NOTE: Read the operating instructions so you understand exactly how the thermometer must be used.

2. Wash hands. Put on gloves if needed.

   CAUTION: Follow standard precautions if contact with open sores or body fluids is possible.

3. Introduce yourself. Identify the patient. Explain the procedure.

4. Remove the thermometer from its base.

5. Install a probe cover according to instructions. This will usually activate the thermometer, showing the word *ready*, indicating the thermometer is ready for use.

   CAUTION: Do not use the thermometer until *ready* is displayed because inaccurate readings will result.

6. Position the patient. Infants under 1 year of age should be positioned lying flat with the head turned for easy access to the ear. Small children can be held on the parent's lap, with the head held against the parent's chest for support. Adults who can cooperate and hold the head steady can either sit or lie flat. Patients in bed should have the head turned to the side and stabilized against the pillow.

7. Hold the thermometer in your right hand to take a temperature in the right ear and in your left hand to take a temperature in the left ear. With your other hand, pull the ear pinna (external lobe) up and back on any child over 1 year of age and on adults. Pull the ear pinna straight back for infants under 1 year of age.

   NOTE: Pulling the pinna correctly straightens the auditory canal so the probe tip will point directly at the tympanic membrane.

8. Insert the covered probe into the ear canal as far as possible to seal the canal.

9. Hold the thermometer steady and press the scan or activation button. Hold it for the required amount of time, usually 1 to 2 seconds, until the reading is displayed on the screen.

10. Remove the thermometer from the patient's ear. Read and record the temperature. Place a (T) by the recording to indicate tympanic temperature.

    NOTE: The temperature will remain on the screen until the probe cover is removed.

    CAUTION: If the temperature reading is low or does not appear to be accurate, change the probe cover and repeat the procedure. The opposite ear can be used for comparison.

11. Press the eject button on the thermometer to discard the probe cover into a waste container.

12. Return the thermometer to its base.

13. Reposition the patient. Observe all safety checkpoints before leaving the patient.

14. Remove gloves and discard in an infectious waste container. Wash hands.

15. Record required information on the patient's chart or agency form, for example, date and time, T 98° (T), your signature and title. Report any abnormal reading to your supervisor immediately.

Procedure 12:2C (cont.)

Practice *Use the evaluation sheet for 12:2C, Measuring and Recording Tympanic (Aural) Temperature, to practice this procedure. When you feel you have mastered this skill, sign the sheet and give it to your instructor for further action.*

✔**Final Checkpoint** Using the criteria listed on the evaluation sheet, your instructor will grade your performance.

Name _____ Date _____

Evaluated by _____

DIRECTIONS: Practice measuring and recording a tympanic (aural) temperature according to the criteria listed. When you are ready for your final check, give this sheet to your instructor.

Measuring and Recording Tympanic (Aural) Temperature	Points Possible	Yes	No	Points Earned	Comments
1. Assembles equipment and supplies	3				
2. Washes hands and puts on gloves if needed	4				
3. Introduces self and identifies patient	4				
4. Explains procedure	4				
5. Removes thermometer from base	5				
6. Installs probe cover correctly	5				
7. Checks that thermometer indicates "ready"	5				
8. Positions patient correctly with easy access to ear	4				
9. Pulls ear pinna back:					
Pulls straight back for infant under 1 year	4				
Pulls up and back for children and adults	4				
10. Inserts probe into ear canal and seals canal	5				
11. Presses scan or activation button	5				
12. Holds thermometer steady for 1 or 2 seconds or time required	5				
13. Removes probe from ear	5				
14. Reads temperature correctly	7				
15. Records correctly and places (T) by reading	7				
16. Removes and discards probe cover correctly	4				
17. Returns thermometer to base unit	4				
18. Repositions patient for comfort and safety	4				
19. Replaces all equipment	3				
20. Removes gloves if worn and washes hands	4				
21. Recognizes an abnormal reading and reports it immediately	5				
Totals	100				

ASSIGNMENT SHEET

Grade _____ Name _____

INTRODUCTION: One of the vital signs you will be required to record is pulse. This assignment sheet will assist you in learning the sites for taking pulse and the important aspects about pulse.

INSTRUCTIONS: Read the information on Measuring and Recording Pulse. In the space provided, print the word(s) that best completes the statement or answers the question.

1. Define *pulse*.

2. a. Study the outlined figure. As you identify each pulse site, enter the name beside the corresponding letter on the following list.

   A.

   B.

   C.

   D.

   E.

   F.

   G.

   b. Circle the site (on the sketch) that is used most frequently for taking pulse.

3. The three (3) factors that must be noted about each and every pulse are:

4. What is the normal pulse range for each of the following?

   a. adults:

   b. children over 7 years old:

   c. children from 1 to 7 years old:

   d. infants:

5. List two (2) factors that could cause an increase in a pulse rate.

6. List two (2) factors that could cause a decrease in a pulse rate.

7. In an adult, a pulse rate under 60 beats per minute is called _____. A pulse rate above 100 beats per minute is called _____. An irregular or abnormal rhythm is a/an _____.

PROCEDURE 12:3 MEASURING AND RECORDING RADIAL PULSE

Equipment and Supplies

Watch with second hand, paper, pencil/pen

Procedure

1. Assemble equipment.

2. Wash hands.

3. Introduce yourself. Identify the patient. Explain the procedure.

4. Place the patient in a comfortable position, with the arm supported and the palm of the hand turned downward.
   NOTE: If the forearm rests on the chest, it will be easier to count respirations after taking the pulse.

5. With the tips of your first two or three fingers, locate the pulse on the thumb side of the patient's wrist.
   NOTE: Do not use your thumb; use your fingers. The thumb contains a pulse that you may confuse with the patient's pulse.

6. When the pulse is felt, exert slight pressure and start counting. Use the second hand of the watch and count for 1 full minute.
   NOTE: In some agencies, the pulse is counted for 30 seconds. The final number is then multiplied by 2. To detect irregularities, it is better to count for 1 full minute.

7. Note the volume (character or strength) and the rhythm (regularity) while counting the pulse.

8. Record the following information: date, time, rate, rhythm, and volume. Follow your agency's policy for recording.

9. Check the patient before leaving. Observe all safety precautions to protect the patient.

10. Replace all equipment used.

11. Wash hands.

12. Record all required information on the patient's chart or agency form, for example, date, time, P 82 strong and regular, your signature and title. Report any unusual observations to your supervisor immediately.

Practice *Use the evaluation sheet for 12:3, Measuring and Recording Radial Pulse, to practice this procedure. When you feel you have mastered this skill, sign the sheet and give it to your instructor for further action.*

✔**Final Checkpoint** Using the criteria listed on the evaluation sheet, your instructor will grade your performance.

12:3 EVALUATION SHEET

Name _____ Date _____

Evaluated by _____

DIRECTIONS: Practice measuring and recording radial pulse according to the criteria listed. When you are ready for your final check, give this sheet to your instructor.

Measuring and Recording Radial Pulse	Points Possible	Yes	No	Points Earned	Comments
1. Assembles supplies	5				
2. Washes hands	5				
3. Introduces self, identifies patient, and explains procedure	6				
4. Positions patient with arm supported and palm down	8				
5. Places finger correctly over selected pulse site	8				
6. Counts 1 minute	8				
7. Obtains correct count to ±2 beats per minute	15				
8. Records accurately	10				
9. Notes rhythm and volume	10				
10. Checks patient before leaving	6				
11. Replaces equipment	5				
12. Washes hands	5				
13. Recognizes an abnormal measurement and reports it immediately	9				
Totals	100				

12:4 MEASURING AND RECORDING RESPIRATIONS

ASSIGNMENT SHEET

Grade _____ Name _____

INTRODUCTION: This assignment will help you review the main facts regarding respirations.

INSTRUCTIONS: Read the information on Measuring and Recording Respirations. In the space provided, print the word(s) that best completes the statement or answers the question.

1. Define *respiration*.

2. One respiration consists of one _____ and one _____.

3. What is the normal rate for respirations in adults?

   What is the normal rate for children?

   What is the normal rate for infants?

4. List three (3) words to describe the character or volume of respirations.

5. List two (2) words to describe the rhythm of respirations.

6. Briefly define the following words.

   dyspnea:

   apnea:

   Cheyne–Stokes:

   rales:

   tachypnea:

   bradypnea:

   wheezing:

7. Why is it important that the patient is not aware that you are counting respirations?

8. If you are taking a TPR, how can you count respirations without letting the patient know that you are doing it?

Equipment and Supplies

Watch with second hand, paper, pen/pencil

Procedure

1. Assemble equipment.

2. Wash hands.

3. Introduce yourself. Identify the patient.

4. After the pulse rate has been counted, leave your hand in position on the pulse site. Count the number of times the chest rises and falls during one minute.

   NOTE: This is done so the patient is not aware that respirations are being counted. If patients are aware, they can change their rate of breathing.

5. Count each expiration and inspiration as one respiration.

6. Note the depth (character) and rhythm (regularity) of the respirations.

7. Record the following information: date, time, rate, character, and rhythm.

8. Check the patient before leaving the area. Observe all safety precautions to protect the patient.

9. Replace all equipment.

10. Wash hands.

11. Record all required information on the patient's chart or agency form, for example, date, time, R 16 deep and regular (or even), your signature and title. Report any unusual observations to your supervisor immediately.

Practice *Use the evaluation sheet for 12:4, Measuring and Recording Respirations, to practice this procedure. When you feel you have mastered this skill, sign the sheet and give it to your instructor for further action.*

✔ **Final Checkpoint** Using the criteria listed on the evaluation sheet, your instructor will grade your performance.

Name _____ Date _____

Evaluated by _____

DIRECTIONS: Practice measuring and recording respirations according to the criteria listed. When you are ready for your final check, give this sheet to your instructor.

Measuring and Recording Respirations	Points Possible	Yes	No	Points Earned	Comments
1. Assembles supplies	5				
2. Washes hands	5				
3. Introduces self and identifies patient	5				
4. Positions patient correctly	5				
5. Leaves hand on pulse site	7				
6. Counts 1 minute	7				
7. Keeps patient unaware of counting activity	8				
8. Obtains correct count to ±1 breath per minute	15				
9. Records correctly	10				
10. Notes rhythm and character	10				
11. Checks patient before leaving	5				
12. Replaces equipment	5				
13. Washes hands	5				
14. Recognizes an abnormal measurement and reports it immediately	8				
Totals	100				

12:5 MEASURING AND RECORDING APICAL PULSE

ASSIGNMENT SHEET

Grade _____ Name _____

INTRODUCTION: The following assignment will help you review the main facts regarding apical pulse.

INSTRUCTIONS: Read the information on Measuring and Recording Apical Pulse. In the space provided, print the word(s) that best answers the question.

1. Define *apical pulse.*

2. List two (2) diseases or conditions a patient may have that would require that an apical pulse be taken.

3. Why are apical pulses usually taken on infants and children?

4. What causes the lubb-dupp heart sounds that are heard while taking an apical pulse?

5. What should you do if you hear any abnormal sounds or beats while taking an apical pulse?

6. What causes a pulse deficit or a higher rate for an apical pulse than for a radial pulse?

7. Calculate the pulse deficit for the following readings.

   Apical pulse 104, radial pulse 80:

   Apical pulse 142, radial pulse 96:

   Apical pulse 86, radial pulse 86:

8. How is the stethoscope cleaned before and after an apical pulse is taken?

Equipment and Supplies

Stethoscope, watch with second hand, paper, pencil/pen, alcohol or disinfectant swab

Procedure

1. Assemble equipment. Use alcohol or a disinfectant to wipe the earpieces and the bell/diaphragm of the stethoscope.

2. Wash hands.

3. Introduce yourself. Identify the patient and explain the procedure. If the patient is an infant or child, explain the procedure to the parent(s).

    NOTE: It is usually best to say, "I am going to listen to your heartbeat." Some patients do not know what an apical pulse is.

4. Close the door to the room. Screen the unit or draw curtains around the bed to provide privacy.

5. Uncover the left side of the patient's chest. The stethoscope must be placed directly against the skin.

6. Place the stethoscope tips in your ears. Locate the apex of the heart, 2 to 3 inches to the left of the breastbone. Use your index finger to locate the fifth intercostal (between the ribs) space at the midclavicular (collarbone) line. Place the bell/diaphragm over the apical region and listen for heart sounds.

    CAUTION: Be sure the tips of the stethoscope are facing forward before placing them in your ears.

7. Count the apical pulse for 1 full minute. Note the rate, rhythm, and volume.

    NOTE: Remember to count each lubb-dupp as one beat.

8. If you doubt your count, recheck your count for another minute.

9. Record your reading. Note date, time, rate, rhythm, and volume. Chart according to the agency policy. Some use an *A* and others use an *AP* to denote apical pulse.

    NOTE: If both a radial and apical pulse are taken, they may be recorded as A82/R82. If a pulse deficit exists, it should be noted. For example, with A80/R64, there is a pulse deficit of 16 (that is, 80 − 64 = 16). This would be recorded as A80/R64 Pulse deficit: 16.

10. Check all safety and comfort points before leaving the patient.

11. Use an alcohol or disinfectant swab to clean the earpieces and the bell/diaphragm of the stethoscope. Replace all equipment.

12. Wash hands.

13. Record all required information on the patient's chart or agency form. For example: date, time, AP 86 strong and regular, your signature and title. If any abnormalities or changes were observed, note and report these immediately.

Practice *Use the evaluation sheet for 12:5, Measuring and Recording Apical Pulse, to practice this procedure. When you feel you have mastered this skill, sign the sheet and give it to your instructor for further action.*

✔ **Final Checkpoint** Using the criteria listed on the evaluation sheet, your instructor will grade your performance.

12:5 Evaluation Sheet

Name _____ Date _____

Evaluated by _____

DIRECTIONS: Practice measuring and recording an apical pulse according to the criteria listed. When you are ready for your final check, give this sheet to your instructor.

Measuring and Recording Apical Pulse	Points Possible	Yes	No	Points Earned	Comments
1. Assembles equipment and supplies. Cleans earpieces and bell/diaphragm with disinfectant	5				
2. Washes hands	5				
3. Introduces self, identifies patient, and explains procedure	5				
4. Avoids unnecessary exposure of patient	6				
5. Places stethoscope in ears properly	7				
6. Places stethoscope on apical area	7				
7. Counts 1 full minute	7				
8. Obtains pulse count accurate to ±2 beats per minute	15				
9. Notes rhythm and volume of pulse	10				
10. Records apical pulse information correctly	10				
11. Checks patient before leaving	6				
12. Cleans and replaces equipment	5				
13. Washes hands	5				
14. Recognizes an abnormal measurement and reports it immediately	7				
Totals	100				

12:6 MEASURING AND RECORDING BLOOD PRESSURE

ASSIGNMENT SHEET 1

Grade _____ Name _____

INTRODUCTION: The following assignment will help you review the main facts regarding blood pressure.

INSTRUCTIONS: Read the information on Measuring and Recording Blood Pressure. Then answer the following questions in the spaces provided.

1. Define *blood pressure.*

2. Define *systolic.*

3. Define *diastolic.*

4. The average reading for systolic pressure is _____ with a range of _____.

5. The average reading for diastolic pressure is _____ with a range of _____.

6. What is the pulse pressure if the blood pressure is 136/72?

7. Hypertension is indicated when pressures are greater than _____ systolic and _____ diastolic.

8. List three (3) causes of hypotension.

9. What is orthostatic, or postural, hypotension? What causes it?

10. List three (3) factors that can increase blood pressure.

11. List three (3) factors that can decrease or lower blood pressure.

12. Why does OSHA discourage the use of mercury sphygmomanometers?

13. a. Record the following blood pressure readings correctly.

Systolic	128	Diastolic	92
Diastolic	84	Systolic	188
Systolic	136	Diastolic	76
Diastolic	118	Systolic	210

b. Name all the above readings that fall within normal range.

c. Name the above readings that do not fall within normal range.

14. Why is it important to use the correct size cuff?

ASSIGNMENT SHEET 2

Grade _____   Name _____

INTRODUCTION: The mercury gauge is a long column. Each mark represents 2 mm Hg. Complete this assignment sheet to learn how to record readings from this mercury gauge.

INSTRUCTIONS: In the space provided, place the reading to which the arrow is pointing.

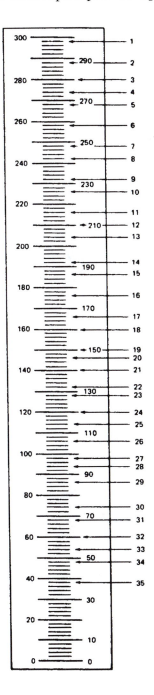

1. _____
2. _____
3. _____
4. _____
5. _____
6. _____
7. _____
8. _____
9. _____
10. _____
11. _____
12. _____
13. _____
14. _____
15. _____
16. _____
17. _____
18. _____
19. _____
20. _____
21. _____
22. _____
23. _____
24. _____
25. _____
26. _____
27. _____
28. _____
29. _____
30. _____
31. _____
32. _____
33. _____
34. _____
35. _____

ASSIGNMENT SHEET 3

Grade _____ Name _____

INTRODUCTION: The aneroid gauge is a common gauge on many sphygmomanometers. Each line represents 2 mm Hg pressure. Complete this sheet to practice reading the gauge.

INSTRUCTIONS: In the spaces provided, place the reading to which the arrow is pointing.

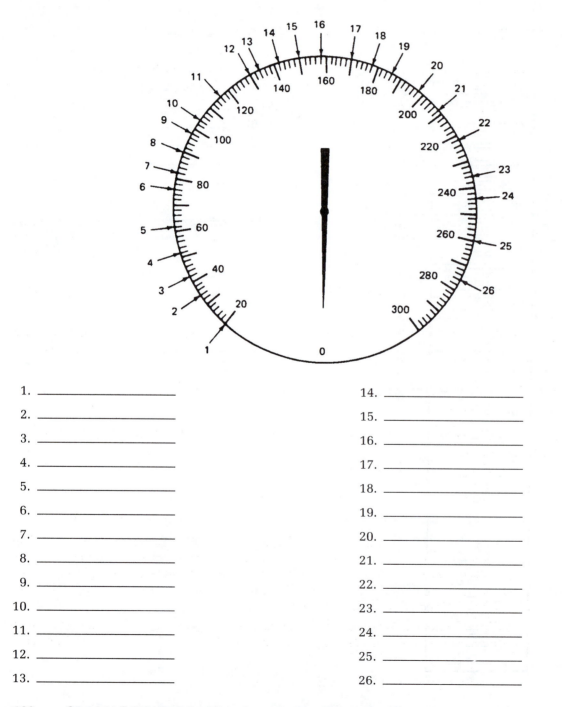

1. _____   14. _____

2. _____   15. _____

3. _____   16. _____

4. _____   17. _____

5. _____   18. _____

6. _____   19. _____

7. _____   20. _____

8. _____   21. _____

9. _____   22. _____

10. _____   23. _____

11. _____   24. _____

12. _____   25. _____

13. _____   26. _____

PROCEDURE 12:6 MEASURING AND RECORDING BLOOD PRESSURE

Equipment and Supplies

Stethoscope, sphygmomanometer, alcohol swab or disinfectant, paper, pencil/pen

Procedure

1. Assemble equipment. Use an alcohol swab or disinfectant to clean the earpieces and bell/diaphragm of the stethoscope.

2. Wash hands.

3. Introduce yourself. Identify the patient. Explain the procedure.

   NOTE: If possible, allow the patient to sit quietly for 5 minutes before taking the blood pressure.

   NOTE: Reassure the patient as needed. Nervous tension and excitement can alter or elevate blood pressure.

4. Roll up the patient's sleeve to approximately 5 inches above the elbow. Position the arm so that it is supported, comfortable, and close to the level of the heart. The palm should be up.

   NOTE: If the sleeve constricts the arm, remove the garment. The arm must be bare and unconstricted for an accurate reading.

5. Wrap the deflated cuff around the upper arm 1 to 1½ inches above the elbow and over the brachial artery. The center of the bladder inside the cuff should be over the brachial artery.

   CAUTION: Do not pull the cuff too tight. The cuff should be smooth and even.

6. Determine the palpatory systolic pressure. To do this, find the radial pulse and keep your fingers on it. Inflate the cuff until the radial pulse disappears. Inflate the cuff 30 mm Hg above this point. Slowly release the pressure on the cuff while watching the gauge. When the pulse is felt again, note the reading on the gauge. This is the palpatory systolic pressure.

7. Deflate the cuff completely. Ask the patient to raise the arm and flex the fingers to promote blood flow. Wait 30 to 60 seconds to allow blood flow to resume completely.

8. Use your fingertips to locate the brachial artery. The brachial artery is located on the inner part of the arm at the antecubital space (area where the elbow bends). Place the stethoscope over the artery. Put the earpieces in your ears.

   NOTE: Earpieces should be pointed forward.

9. Check to make sure the tubings are separate and not tangled together.

10. Gently close the valve on the rubber bulb by turning it in a clockwise direction. Inflate the cuff to 30 mm Hg above the palpatory systolic pressure.

    NOTE: Make sure the sphygmomanometer gauge is at eye level.

11. Open the bulb valve slowly and let the air escape gradually.

12. When the first sound is heard, note the reading on the manometer. This is the systolic pressure.

13. Continue to release the air until there is an abrupt change of the sound, usually soft or muffled. Note the reading on the manometer. Continue to release the air until the sound changes again, becoming first faint and then no longer heard. Note the reading on the manometer. The point at which the first change in sound occurs is the diastolic pressure in children. The diastolic pressure in adults is the point at which the sound becomes very faint or stops.

    NOTE: If you still hear sound, continue to the zero mark. Record both readings (the change of sound and the zero reading). For a systolic of 122 and a continued diastolic of 78, this can be written as 122/78/0.

14. When the sound ceases, rapidly deflate the cuff.

Procedure 12:6 (cont.)

15. If you need to repeat the procedure to recheck your reading, completely deflate the cuff. Wait 1 minute before repeating the procedure. Ask the patient to raise the arm and flex the fingers to promote blood flow.

> **!** **CAUTION:** If you cannot obtain a reading, report to your supervisor promptly.

16. Record the time and your reading. The reading is written as a fraction, with systolic over diastolic. For example, BP 124/72 (or 124/80/72 if the change in sound is noted).

17. Remove the cuff. Expel any remaining air by squeezing the cuff. Use alcohol or a disinfectant to clean the stethoscope earpieces and diaphragm/bell. Replace all equipment.

18. Check patient for safety and comfort before leaving.

19. Wash hands.

20. Record all required information on the patient's chart or agency form, for example, date, time, BP 126/74, your signature and title. Report any abnormal readings to your supervisor immediately.

Practice *Use the evaluation sheet for 12:6, Measuring and Recording Blood Pressure, to practice this procedure. When you feel you have mastered this skill, sign the sheet and give it to your instructor for further action.*

✔ **Final Checkpoint** Using the criteria listed on the evaluation sheet, your instructor will grade your performance.

Name _____ Date _____

Evaluated by _____

DIRECTIONS: Practice measuring and recording blood pressure according to the criteria listed. When you are ready for your final check, give this sheet to your instructor.

Measuring and Recording Blood Pressure	Points Possible	Yes	No	Points Earned	Comments
1. Assembles equipment and supplies. Cleans stethoscope earpieces and and bell/disk with a disinfectant	3				
2. Washes hands	3				
3. Introduces self and identifies patient	3				
4. Explains procedure	3				
5. Uses correct size cuff and applies it correctly	4				
6. Determines palpatory systolic pressure	4				
7. Deflates cuff and waits 30–60 seconds	4				
8. Places stethoscope in ears correctly	4				
9. Locates brachial artery	4				
10. Inflates cuff 30 mm Hg above palpatory systolic pressure	4				
11. Uses aneroid sphygmomanometer:					
Places gauge correctly	4				
Untangles tubing	4				
Reads pressure to ±2 mm Hg	8				
Records correctly	4				
12. Uses mercury sphygmomanometer:					
Sets on flat surface	4				
Reads to ±2 mm Hg	8				
Records correctly	4				
13. Reads adult diastolic as cessation of sound	5				
14. Reads child diastolic as change in sound	5				
15. Checks patient for comfort and safety	4				
16. Cleans stethoscope earpieces and bell/disk with a disinfectant	4				
17. Replaces equipment	3				
18. Washes hands	3				
19. Recognizes an abnormal measurement and reports it immediately	4				
Totals	100				

CHAPTER 12 INTERNET SEARCHES

Use the suggested search engines in Chapter 9:4 of the textbook to search the Internet for additional information on the following topics:

1. *Organization:* Find the American Heart Association web site to obtain information on the heart, pulse, arrhythmias, and blood pressure.

2. *Vital signs:* Research body temperature, pulse, respiration, blood pressure, and apical pulse.

3. *Temperature scales:* Research Celsius (centigrade) versus Fahrenheit temperatures. Try to locate conversion charts that can be used to compare the two scales.

4. *Diseases:* Research hypothermia, fever or pyrexia, hypertension, hypotension, and heart arrhythmias.

CHAPTER 13 FIRST AID

13:1 PROVIDING FIRST AID

ASSIGNMENT SHEET

Grade _____ Name _____

INTRODUCTION: The following assignment will help you review the main facts on general guidelines for first aid.

INSTRUCTIONS: Study the information on Providing First Aid. In the space provided, print the word(s) that best answers the question or completes the statement.

1. Define *first aid*.

2. The type of first aid treatment you provide will vary depending on several factors. List two (2) factors that may affect any action taken.

3. Identify three (3) senses that can alert you to an emergency.

4. What action should you take if you notice that it is not safe to approach the scene of an accident?

5. What is the first thing you should determine when you get to the victim?

6. Why is it important to avoid moving a victim whenever possible?

7. List four (4) kinds of information that should be reported while calling emergency medical services (EMS).

8. What should you do if a person refuses to give consent for care?

9. What is triage?

10. Identify four (4) life-threatening emergencies that must be cared for first.

11. List two (2) sources of information you can use to find out the details regarding an accident, injury, or illness.

12. Why shouldn't you discuss the victim's condition with observers at the scene?

13. While providing first aid to the victim, make every attempt to avoid further _____.
    Provide only the treatment you are _____ to provide.

13:2 PERFORMING CARDIOPULMONARY RESUSCITATION (CPR)

ASSIGNMENT SHEET

Grade _____ Name _____

INTRODUCTION: This assignment will help you review the main facts regarding CPR.

INSTRUCTIONS: Review the information on Performing Cardiopulmonary Resuscitation (CPR). In the space provided, print the word(s) that best completes the statement or answers the question.

1. CPR stands for _____.

2. What do the ABCDs of CPR represent?

3. How does biological death differ from clinical death?

4. When does biological death occur?

5. What two (2) methods can be used to open the airway?

6. What is an AED? How is it used?

7. What should you determine first before starting CPR?

8. Identify each of the following situations as either a "call first" or "call fast" emergency.

   a. any victim of submersion or near-drowning:

   b. an unconscious adult or child 8-years-old or older:

   c. an unconscious infant with a high risk for heart problems:

   d. an unconscious infant or child less than 8-years-old:

   e. any victim with cardiac arrest caused by trauma or a drug overdose:

9. What is the three-point evaluation that is used to check for breathing?

10. What pulse site is checked to determine whether compression is necessary on an adult?

11. To perform a one-person rescue on an adult victim, give _____ compressions followed by _____ respirations. Compressions are given at the rate of _____ per minute. _____ 15:2 cycles should be completed every minute. Pressure should be applied straight down to compress the sternum about _____ inches or _____ centimeters.

12. To rescue an infant, both the infant's _____ and _____ are covered for ventilations. Two fingers are placed on the sternum _____ below a line drawn between the nipples, and the sternum is compressed _____ inches or _____ centimeters. Compressions are given at the rate of at least _____ per minute. After each _____ compressions, give one ventilation for a ratio of _____:_____ compressions to ventilations.

13. CPR for a child is used when the child is under 8 years of age. Compressions are given at the rate of _____ per minute. The heel of one hand is placed on the sternum _____ above the _____. The sternum is compressed _____ inches or _____ centimeters. The ratio of compressions to ventilations is _____:_____.

14. What should you do for a choking victim who is conscious, coughing, and able to breathe?

15. Briefly list the sequence of steps used to remove an obstruction in an unconscious adult victim who has an obstructed airway.

16. Briefly list the sequence of steps used to remove an obstruction in an infant with an obstructed airway.

17. You have tried to remove an obstruction from an airway for several minutes, but the airway is still blocked. Should you check the pulse and start chest compressions at this point? Why or why not?

18. List four (4) reasons for stopping CPR once it is started.

PROCEDURE 13:2A PERFORMING CPR—ONE-PERSON RESCUE

Equipment and Supplies

CPR manikin, alcohol or disinfecting solution, gauze sponges

Procedure

⚠ **CAUTION:** Only a CPR training manikin should be used to practice this procedure. *Never* practice CPR on another person.

1. Assemble equipment. Position the manikin on a firm surface, usually the floor.

2. Check for consciousness. Shake the "victim" by tapping the shoulder. Ask, "Are you OK?" If the victim does not respond, activate EMS immediately. Follow the "call first, call fast" priority.

3. Open the airway. Use the head-tilt/chin-lift method. Place one hand on the victim's forehead. Place the fingertips of the other hand under the bony part of the victim's jaw, near the chin. Tilt the head without closing the victim's mouth.

   NOTE: This action moves the tongue away from the back of the throat and prevents the tongue from blocking the airway.

   ⚠ **CAUTION:** If the victim has a suspected neck or upper spinal cord injury, use a jaw-thrust maneuver to open the airway. Grasp the angles of the victim's lower jaw by positioning one hand on each side. Lift with both hands to move the lower jaw forward, making every attempt to avoid excessive backward tilting or side-to-side movement of the head.

4. Check for breathing. Put your ear close to the victim's nose and mouth while looking at the chest. Look, listen, and feel for respirations for about 5 but not more than 10 seconds.

5. *If the victim is breathing*, keep the airway open and obtain medical help. *If the victim is not breathing*, administer mouth-to-mouth resuscitation as follows:

   a. Keep the airway open.

   b. Resting your hand on the victim's forehead, use your thumb and forefinger to pinch the victim's nose shut.

   c. Seal the victim's mouth with your mouth.

   d. Give 2 slow breaths, each lasting approximately 2 seconds until the chest rises gently. Pause slightly between breaths. This allows air to flow out and provides you with a chance to take a breath and increase the oxygen level for the second rescue breath.

   e. Watch the chest for movement to be sure the air is entering the victim's lungs. Avoid overinflating the lungs and/or forcing air into the stomach.

    CAUTION: Follow standard precautions. If possible, use a CPR pocket face mask with a one-way valve to provide a barrier and prevent the transmission of disease.

6. *Palpate the carotid pulse:* Kneeling at the victim's side, place the fingertips of your hand on the victim's voice box. Then slide the fingers toward you and into the groove at the side of the victim's neck, where you should find the carotid pulse. Take at least 5 seconds but not more than 10 seconds to feel for the pulse. At the same time, watch for breathing, signs of circulation, and/or movement.

   NOTE: The pulse may be weak, so check carefully.

7. *If the victim has a pulse*, continue providing mouth-to-mouth resuscitation. Give one slow, gentle breath every 5 seconds. Count, "One, one thousand; two, one thousand; three, one thousand; four, one thousand; and breathe," to obtain the correct timing. After 1 minute of rescue breathing (approximately 12 breaths), recheck the pulse to make sure the heart is still beating.

8. *If the victim does not have a pulse*, administer chest compressions as follows:

   a. Locate the correct place on the sternum. While kneeling alongside the victim, use the middle finger of your hand that is closest to the victim's feet to follow the ribs up to where the ribs meet the sternum, at the substernal notch. Keep the middle finger on the notch and position the index finger

Procedure 13:2A (cont.)

above it so two fingers are on the sternum. Then, place the heel of the opposite hand (the one closest to the victim's head) on the sternum, next to the index finger.

CAUTION: The heel of your hand should be approximately 1 to 1½ inches above the end of the sternum.

b. Place your other hand on top of the hand that is correctly positioned. Keep your fingers off the victim's chest. It may help to interlock your fingers.

c. Rise up on your knees so that your shoulders are directly over the victim's sternum. Lock your elbows and keep your arms straight.
NOTE: This position will allow you to push straight down on the sternum and compress the heart, which lies between the sternum and vertebral column.

d. Push straight down to compress the chest approximately 1½ to 2 inches, or 3.8 to 5.0 centimeters. Use a smooth, even motion.

e. Administer 15 compressions at the rate of 100 per minute. Count, "One and, two and, three and," and so forth, to obtain the correct rate.

f. Allow the chest to relax completely after each compression. Keep your hands on the sternum during the upstroke (chest relaxation period).

g. The 15 compressions should be completed in approximately 10 seconds.

9. After administering 15 compressions, give the victim 2 ventilations, or breaths. Avoid excessive body movement while giving the ventilations. Keep your knees in the same position and swing your body upward to give the respirations. Respirations should be completed in approximately 5 seconds.

10. Repeat the cycle of 15 compressions followed by 2 ventilations. After four cycles of a 15:2 ratio, take 5 seconds to check the victim for breathing and the presence of a carotid pulse. If no pulse is felt, continue providing 15 compressions followed by 2 respirations.
NOTE: Remember, cardiac compressions are applied only if the victim has no pulse.

11. After you begin CPR, do not stop unless
a. The victim recovers.
b. Help arrives to take over and give CPR and/or apply an AED.
c. A physician or other legally qualified person orders you to discontinue the attempt.
d. You are so physically exhausted, you cannot continue.
e. The scene suddenly becomes unsafe.
f. You are given a legally valid do not resuscitate (DNR) order.

12. After the practice session, use a gauze pad saturated with 70 percent alcohol or a 10 percent bleach disinfecting solution to clean the manikin. Wipe the face and clean inside the mouth thoroughly. Saturate a clean gauze pad with the solution and lay it on the mouth area for at least 30 seconds. Use another gauze pad to wipe the area dry. Follow manufacturer's instructions for any additional cleaning required.
NOTE: A 10 percent bleach solution is more effective than alcohol. Some manikins have disposable mouthpieces that are discarded after use. If the mouthpiece is discarded, the remainder of the face should still be disinfected.

13. Replace all equipment used. Wash hands.

Practice *Use the evaluation sheet for 13:2A, Performing CPR—One-Person Rescue, to practice this procedure. When you feel you have mastered this skill, sign the sheet and give it to your instructor for further action.*

✔ **Final Checkpoint** Using the criteria listed on the evaluation sheet, your instructor will grade your performance.

Name _____ Date _____

Evaluated by _____

DIRECTIONS: Practice performing CPR (cardiopulmonary resuscitation) with a one-person rescue according to the criteria listed. When you are ready for your final check, give this sheet to your instructor.

Performing CPR—One-Person Rescue	Points Possible	Yes	No	Points Earned	Comments
1. Assembles equipment and supplies and places manikin on firm surface	1				
2. Checks consciousness:					
Shakes victim by tapping shoulder	3				
Asks "Are you OK?"	3				
3. If the victim is unconscious, follows "call first, call fast" priorities	5				
4. Opens airway with head-tilt/chin-lift method or jaw-thrust maneuver if victim has suspected neck or spine injury	5				
5. Looks, listens, and feels for respirations for 5 but not more than 10 seconds	5				
6. Gives 2 slow breaths until the chest rises gently	5				
7. Palpates carotid pulse for 5 but not more than 10 seconds	5				
8. Administers chest compressions as follows:					
Locates correct hand position on sternum	5				
Places heel of hands on chest with fingers off of chest	5				
Positions shoulders above sternum to apply vertical force	5				
Keeps elbows straight	5				
Compresses 1½ to 2 inches	5				
Gives 15 compressions at rate of 100 per minute	5				
Counts "one and, two and . . . "	5				
9. Gives 2 ventilations	5				
10. Repeats cycle of 15 compressions and 2 ventilations giving 4 cycles every minute	5				
11. Checks pulse and breathing for 5 but not more than 10 seconds after 4 cycles	5				
12. Resumes CPR by giving 2 breaths and then continues 15:2 cycle	5				
13. Continues CPR until:					
Victim recovers	2				
Qualified help takes over	2				
Physician orders attempt discontinued	2				
Too physically exhausted	2				
Scene suddenly becomes unsafe	2				
Presented with a valid DNR order	2				
14. Cleans and replaces all equipment used	1				
Totals	100				

PROCEDURE 13:2B PERFORMING CPR ON INFANTS

Equipment and Supplies

CPR infant manikin, alcohol or disinfecting solution, gauze pads

Procedure

(!) CAUTION: Only a CPR training manikin should be used to practice this procedure. *Never* practice CPR on a human infant.

1. Assemble equipment.

2. Gently shake the infant or tap the infant's foot (for reflex action) to determine consciousness. Call to the infant.

3. If the infant is unconscious, call aloud for help and begin the steps of CPR. If no one arrives to call EMS, stop CPR after 1 minute to telephone for medical assistance. Resume CPR as quickly as possible.

   NOTE: If the infant is known to have a high risk for heart problems, call first and then begin CPR.

4. Use the head-tilt/chin-lift method to open the infant's airway. Tip the head back gently, taking care not to tip it as far back as you would an adult's head.

   (!) CAUTION: Tipping the head too far will cause an obstruction of the infant's airway.

   NOTE: For CPR techniques, infants are usually considered to be under 1 year old.

5. Look, listen, and feel for breathing. Check for at least 5 but not more than 10 seconds.

6. *If there is no breathing*, give 2 slow, gentle breaths, each breath lasting approximately 1½ seconds. Cover the infant's nose and mouth with your mouth. Breathe until the chest rises gently during each ventilation. Allow for chest deflation after each breath.

   (biohazard) CAUTION: Follow standard precautions. If possible, use a CPR pocket face mask with a one-way valve to provide a barrier and prevent the transmission of disease.

7. Check the pulse over the brachial artery. Place your fingertips on the inside of the upper arm and halfway between the elbow and shoulder. Put your thumb on the posterior (outside) of the arm. Squeeze your fingers gently toward your thumb. Feel for the pulse for 5 but not more than 10 seconds.

8. *If a pulse is present*, continue providing ventilations by giving the infant 1 breath every 3 seconds. After 1 minute (approximately 20 breaths), recheck the pulse and breathing for approximately 5 but not more than 10 seconds.

9. *If no pulse is present*, administer cardiac compressions. Locate the correct position for compressions by drawing an imaginary line between the nipples. Place two fingers on the sternum and one finger's width below this imaginary line. Give compressions at the rate of 100 per minute. Make sure the infant is on a firm surface, or use one hand to support the infant's back while administering compressions. Press hard enough to compress the infant's chest ½ to 1 inch, or 1.3 to 2.5 centimeters. Give 5 compressions in approximately 3 seconds.

10. After every 5 compressions, give 1 slow, gentle breath until the chest rises gently.

11. Continue the cycle of 5 compressions followed by 1 ventilation. To establish the correct rate, count, "One, two, three, four, five, breathe."

12. After one minute (about 12 cycles) check for breathing and pulse for approximately 5 but not more than 10 seconds. Continue CPR if no breathing or pulse is noted. Recheck the pulse and breathing every few minutes.

13. After the practice session, use a gauze pad saturated with 70 percent alcohol or a 10 percent bleach disinfecting solution to clean the manikin. Wipe the face and clean inside the mouth thoroughly. Saturate a clean gauze pad with the solution and lay it on the mouth area for at least 30 seconds. Use another gauze pad to wipe the area dry. Follow manufacturer's instructions for specific cleaning.

Procedure 13:2B (cont.)

NOTE: The 10 percent bleach solution is more effective than alcohol. Some manikins have disposable mouthpieces that are discarded after use. If the mouthpiece is discarded, the remainder of the face should still be disinfected.

14. Replace all equipment used. Wash hands.

Practice *Use the evaluation sheet for 13:2B, Performing CPR on Infants, to practice this procedure. When you feel you have mastered this skill, sign the sheet and give it to your instructor for further action.*

✔**Final Checkpoint** Using the criteria listed on the evaluation sheet, your instructor will grade your performance.

Name _____ Date _____

Evaluated by _____

DIRECTIONS: Practice performing CPR (cardiopulmonary resuscitation) on infants according to the criteria listed. When you are ready for your final check, give this sheet to your instructor.

Performing CPR on Infants	Points Possible	Yes	No	Points Earned	Comments
1. Assembles equipment and supplies and places manikin on firm surface	2				
2. Shakes gently and calls to infant	5				
3. Calls aloud for help and follows "call first, call fast" priorities	5				
4. Opens airway but does not tilt head as far back as for an adult	6				
5. Looks, listens, and feels for breathing for 5 but not more than 10 seconds	6				
6. Gives breaths:					
Covers mouth and nose	5				
Gives 2 slow breaths	5				
Watches for chest to rise gently	5				
7. Checks brachial pulse on infants for 5 but not more than 10 seconds	6				
8. Administers compressions:					
Places 2 fingers one finger's width below an imaginary line drawn between the nipples	6				
Gives compressions at rate of 100 per minute	6				
Counts 1, 2, 3, 4, 5, breathe	6				
Compresses ½ to 1 inch or 1.3 to 2.5 centimeters	6				
Supports back or places victim on firm surface	6				
9. Gives 1 ventilation after every 5 compressions	6				
10. Repeats cycle of 5:1 with slight pause for ventilation	6				
11. Checks breathing and pulse after 1 minute—checks for 5 but not more than 10 seconds	6				
12. Continues CPR if no breathing or pulse by starting with one breath	5				
13. Cleans and replaces all equipment	2				
Totals	100				

Equipment and Supplies

CPR child manikin, alcohol or disinfecting solution, gauze pads

Procedure

⚠ **CAUTION:** Only a CPR training manikin should be used to practice this procedure. *Never* practice CPR on a human child.

1. Assemble equipment.

2. Gently shake the child to determine consciousness. Call to the child.

3. If the child is unconscious, call aloud for help and begin the steps of CPR. If no one arrives to call EMS, stop CPR after 1 minute to telephone for medical assistance. Resume CPR as quickly as possible.

   NOTE: If the child is known to have a high risk for heart problems, call first and then begin CPR.

4. Use the head-tilt/chin-lift method to open the child's airway. Tip the head back gently, taking care not to tip it as far back as you would an adult's head.

   NOTE: For CPR techniques, infants are usually considered to be under 1 year old; children are ages 1 to 8 years. Children over 8 years old usually require the same techniques as do adults. Use your judgment for this age group, depending on the size of the child.

5. Look, listen, and feel for breathing. Check for at least 5 but not more than 10 seconds.

6. *If there is no breathing,* give 2 slow, gentle breaths, each breath lasting approximately 1½ seconds. Cover the child's nose and mouth with your mouth, or pinch the child's nose and cover the child's mouth with your mouth. Breathe until the chest rises gently during each ventilation. Allow for chest deflation after each breath.

   ☣ **CAUTION:** Follow standard precautions. If possible, use a CPR pocket face mask with a one-way valve to provide a barrier and prevent the transmission of disease.

7. Check the pulse at the carotid pulse site. Feel for the pulse for 5 but not more than 10 seconds.

8. *If a pulse is present,* continue providing ventilations by giving the child 1 breath every 3 seconds. After 1 minute (approximately 20 breaths), recheck the pulse and breathing for approximately 5 but not more than 10 seconds.

9. *If no pulse is present,* administer cardiac compressions. Place the heel of one hand one finger's width above the substernal notch of the breastbone. Keep the other hand on the child's forehead. Give compressions at the rate of 100 per minute. Make sure the child is on a firm surface, or use one hand to support the child's back while administering compressions. Press hard enough to compress the child's chest 1 to 1½ inches, or 2.5 to 3.8 centimeters. Give 5 compressions in approximately 3 seconds.

10. After every 5 compressions, give 1 slow, gentle breath until the chest rises gently.

11. Continue the cycle of 5 compressions followed by 1 ventilation. To establish the correct rate, count, "One, two, three, four, five, breathe."

12. After one minute (about 12 cycles) check for breathing and pulse for approximately 5 but not more than 10 seconds. Continue CPR if no breathing or pulse is noted. Recheck the pulse and breathing every few minutes.

13. After the practice session, use a gauze pad saturated with 70 percent alcohol or a 10 percent bleach disinfecting solution to clean the manikin. Wipe the face and clean inside the mouth thoroughly. Saturate a clean gauze pad with the solution and lay it on the mouth area for at least 30 seconds. Use another gauze pad to wipe the area dry. Follow manufacturer's instructions for specific cleaning.

    NOTE: The 10 percent bleach solution is more effective than alcohol. Some manikins have disposable mouthpieces that are discarded after use. If the mouthpiece is discarded, the remainder of the face should still be disinfected.

Procedure 13:2C (cont.)

14. Replace all equipment used. Wash hands.

Practice *Use the evaluation sheet for 13:2C, Performing CPR on Children, to practice this procedure. When you feel you have mastered this skill, sign the sheet and give it to your instructor for further action.*

✔ **Final Checkpoint** Using the criteria listed on the evaluation sheet, your instructor will grade your performance.

13:2C EVALUATION SHEET

Name _____ Date _____

Evaluated by _____

DIRECTIONS: Practice performing CPR (cardiopulmonary resuscitation) on children according to the criteria listed. When you are ready for your final check, give this sheet to your instructor.

Performing CPR on Children	Points Possible	Yes	No	Points Earned	Comments
1. Assembles equipment and supplies and places manikin on firm surface	2				
2. Shakes gently and calls to child	5				
3. Obtains medical help as soon as possible following "call first, call fast" priorities	5				
4. Opens airway correctly	6				
5. Looks, listens, and feels for breathing for 5 but not more than 10 seconds	6				
6. Gives breaths:					
Covers nose and mouth or just mouth	5				
Gives 2 slow breaths	5				
Watches for chest to rise	5				
7. Checks carotid pulse for 5 but not more than 10 seconds	6				
8. Administers compressions if no pulse:					
Places heel of one hand one finger's width above substernal notch	6				
Gives compressions at rate of 100 per minute	6				
Counts 1 and 2 and 3 and 4 and 5	6				
Compresses 1–1½ inches or 2.5 to 3.8 centimeters	6				
Supports back or places child on firm surface	6				
9. Gives 1 ventilation after every 5 compressions	6				
10. Repeats cycle of 5:1 with slight pause for ventilations	6				
11. Checks breathing and pulse for 5 but not more than 10 seconds after 1 minute	6				
12. Continues CPR if no breathing or pulse by starting with 1 breath	5				
13. Cleans and replaces all equipment	2				
Totals	100				

Equipment and Supplies

CPR manikin or choking manikin

Procedure

(!) CAUTION: Only a manikin should be used to practice this procedure. Do *not* practice on another person. Hand placement can be tried on another person, but the actual abdominal thrust should *never* be performed unless the person is choking.

1. Assemble equipment. Position the manikin in an upright position sitting on a chair.

2. Determine whether the victim has an airway obstruction. Ask, "Are you choking?" Check to see whether the victim can cough or speak.

   (!) CAUTION: If the victim is coughing, the airway is not completely obstructed. Encourage the victim to remain calm and cough hard. Coughing is usually very effective for removing an obstruction.

3. If the victim cannot cough, talk, make noise, or breathe, call for help.

4. Perform abdominal thrusts to try to remove the obstruction. Follow these steps:

   a. Stand behind the victim.

   b. Wrap both arms around the victim's waist.

   c. Make a fist of one hand. Place the thumb side of the fist in the middle of the victim's abdomen, slightly above the navel (umbilicus) but well below the xiphoid process at the end of the sternum.

   d. Grasp the fist with your other hand.

   e. Use quick, upward thrusts to press into the victim's abdomen.
      NOTE: The thrusts should be delivered hard enough to cause a force of air to push the obstruction out of the airway.
      (!) CAUTION: Make sure that your forearms do not press against the victim's rib cage while the thrusts are being performed.

   f. If you cannot reach around the victim to give abdominal thrusts (the victim is very obese), or if the victim is in the later stages of pregnancy, give chest thrusts. Stand behind the victim. Wrap your arms under the victim's axilla (armpits) and around to the center of the chest. Make a fist with one hand and place the thumb side of the fist against the center of the sternum but well above the xiphoid process. Grab your fist with your other hand and thrust inward.

   g. Repeat the thrusts until the object is expelled or until the victim becomes unconscious. If the victim loses consciousness, follow Procedure 13:2E, Performing CPR—Obstructed Airway on Unconscious Victim. Start with a mouth sweep, try to give 2 breaths, reposition the head and try to give 2 more breaths if the first breaths do not go in, and then give 5 abdominal thrusts if you are unable to ventilate the victim.

5. Make every effort to obtain medical help for the victim as soon as possible. Send someone to call for help. If no one is present, yell for help. If no one answers your calls, you may have to stop your efforts for a short period of time to call EMS.

6. After the practice session, replace all equipment used. Wash hands.

Practice *Use the evaluation sheet for 13:2D, Performing CPR—Obstructed Airway on Conscious Adult Victim, to practice this procedure. When you feel you have mastered this skill, sign the sheet and give it to your instructor for further action.*

✔ **Final Checkpoint** Using the criteria listed on the evaluation sheet, your instructor will grade your performance.

13:2D EVALUATION SHEET

Name _____ Date _____

Evaluated by _____

DIRECTIONS: Practice performing CPR (cardiopulmonary resuscitation) on a conscious adult victim with an obstructed airway according to the criteria listed. When you are ready for your final check, give this sheet to your instructor. **NOTE:** Use only a manikin to perform thrusts.

Performing CPR—Obstructed Airway on Conscious Adult Victim	Points Possible	Yes	No	Points Earned	Comments
1. Assembles equipment and supplies and places manikin in upright position	5				
2. Determines whether victim has an airway obstruction:					
Asks "Are you choking?"	5				
Checks whether victim can cough, talk, or breathe	5				
3. Calls out for help	6				
4. Performs abdominal thrusts:					
Stands behind the victim	8				
Wraps arms around victim's waist	8				
Places thumb side of fist above umbilicus but below xiphoid	8				
Grasps fist with other hand	8				
Uses quick, upward thrusts	8				
5. Demonstrates chest thrusts for very obese or pregnant victim:					
Stands behind victim	4				
Wraps arms under victim's axillae	4				
Places thumb side of fist against center of sternum but well above xiphoid	4				
Grasps fist with other hand	4				
Thrusts inward	4				
6. Repeats thrusts until object expelled or victim loses consciousness	8				
7. Obtains medical help as soon as possible	6				
8. Replaces all equipment	5				
Totals	100				

PROCEDURE 13:2E PERFORMING CPR—OBSTRUCTED AIRWAY ON UNCONSCIOUS VICTIM

Equipment and Supplies

CPR manikin, alcohol or disinfecting solution, gauze sponges

Procedure

CAUTION: Only a manikin should be used to practice this procedure. Do *not* practice on another person.

1. Assemble equipment. Place the manikin on a firm surface, usually the floor.

2. Shake the victim gently. Ask, "Are you OK?"

3. If the victim is unconscious, yell for help. If no one arrives to help, call EMS. If the victim is an infant or child, yell for help, and perform the steps for an unconscious choking victim for approximately 1 minute. If no one arrives to call EMS, stop after 1 minute to call EMS. Resume the steps for an unconscious choking victim as quickly as possible.

4. Use the head-tilt/chin-lift method to open the airway.

5. Look, listen, and feel for breathing for approximately 5 but not more than 10 seconds.

6. If the victim is not breathing, give 2 slow, gentle breaths. If air does not go into the lungs, reposition the victim's head and try to breathe again. If the chest still does not rise, the airway is probably obstructed.

   CAUTION: Follow standard precautions. If possible, use a CPR pocket face mask with a one-way valve to provide a barrier and prevent the transmission of disease.

7. Perform 5 abdominal thrusts. Position the victim on his or her back. Place one of your legs on either side of the hips and thighs and "straddle" the victim. Place the heel of one hand on the victim's abdomen, making sure the heel is positioned well below the tip of the xiphoid process, at the end of the sternum, but slightly above the navel (umbilicus). Place your other hand on top of the first hand. Give 5 quick, upward thrusts into the abdomen.

   NOTE: This action provides a force of air to help free the object obstructing the airway.

   NOTE: If the victim is pregnant or very obese, it may be necessary to give chest thrusts instead of abdominal thrusts. Position your hands in the same position used for chest compressions. Push straight down 5 times.

8. Check the mouth for the object. Open the victim's mouth by grasping the lower jaw between your thumb and fingers and lifting it. This pushes the tongue out of the airway and away from the object that may be lodged there. Use the index finger of your opposite hand to sweep along the inside of the mouth. With a C-shape or hooking motion, bring the finger along one cheek and sweep across the throat from the side and toward the opposite cheek. Remove the object if it is seen.

   CAUTION: Take care not to push straight into the throat because doing so may force the object to lodge deeper in the airway.

9. Open the airway and try to give 2 slow, gentle breaths. If the chest rises, check the pulse and continue with ventilations or CPR as needed.

10. *If the chest does not rise*, reposition the head, and try to breathe again. If the chest still does not rise, repeat the sequence. Give 5 thrusts, check the mouth, and attempt to ventilate. Continue repeating the sequence until you are able to get air into the chest during ventilation.

    NOTE: Unless you are able to get oxygen into the lungs of the victim, chest compressions have no value. The purpose of chest compressions is to circulate the oxygen.

    NOTE: After a period of time without oxygen, the muscles of the throat will relax and you may be able to remove the object using the previous methods.

Procedure 13:2E (cont.)

11. To care for an infant who has an obstructed airway, follow these steps:

   a. Gently shake the infant to determine consciousness. Call to the infant. Call for help if there is no response.

   b. Use the head-tilt/chin-lift method to open the airway.

   c. Look, listen, and feel for breathing for 5 but not more than 10 seconds.

   d. If there is no breathing, cover the infant's nose and mouth with your mouth and attempt to ventilate. If the breaths do not go in, reposition the infant's head and try to breathe a second time. If the breaths still do not go in, assume that the infant has an obstructed airway.

   e. Give 5 back blows. Hold the infant face down, with your arm supporting the infant's body and your hand supporting the infant's head and jaw. Position the head lower than the chest. Use the heel of your other hand to give 5 firm back blows between the infant's shoulder blades.

   CAUTION: When performing back blows on an infant, do not use excessive force.

   f. Give 5 chest thrusts. Turn the infant face up, holding the head lower than the chest. Position two or three fingers on the sternum one finger's width below an imaginary line drawn between the nipples. Gently press straight down 5 times to compress the sternum ½ to 1 inch.

   g. Check the mouth for the object. If you see the object, remove it by using a finger to sweep the mouth.

   CAUTION: If you do *not* see the object, do not sweep the mouth with a finger.

   h. Attempt to ventilate by giving 2 slow breaths. If the infant's chest rises, check for pulse and then continue with pulmonary resuscitation or cardiac compressions, as needed. If the chest does not rise, keep repeating the sequence of 5 back blows, 5 chest thrusts, checking the mouth, and ventilating until the object can be removed.

12. To care for a child who has an obstructed airway, follow the same procedure used for adult victims *except* look in the mouth during the mouth check. Do *not* perform a finger sweep unless the object can be seen in the mouth. The sequence of steps is to give 5 abdominal thrusts, look in the mouth, sweep the mouth if the object is seen, and attempt to ventilate.

13. After the practice session, use a gauze pad saturated with 70 percent alcohol or a 10 percent bleach disinfecting solution to clean the manikin. Wipe the face and clean inside the mouth thoroughly. Saturate a clean gauze pad with the solution and lay it on the mouth area for at least 30 seconds. Use another gauze pad to wipe the area dry. Follow manufacturer's recommendations for specific cleaning or care.

   NOTE: A 10 percent bleach solution is more effective than alcohol. Some manikins have disposable mouthpieces that are discarded after use. If the mouthpiece is discarded, the remainder of the face should still be disinfected.

14. Replace all equipment used. Wash hands.

Practice *Use the evaluation sheet for 13:2E, Performing CPR—Obstructed Airway on Unconscious Victim, to practice this procedure. When you feel you have mastered this skill, sign the sheet and give it to your instructor for further action.*

✔ **Final Checkpoint** Using the criteria listed on the evaluation sheet, your instructor will grade your performance.

13:2E EVALUATION SHEET

Name _____ Date _____

Evaluated by _____

DIRECTIONS: Practice performing CPR (cardiopulmonary resuscitation) on an unconscious victim with an obstructed airway according to the criteria listed. When you are ready for your final check, give this sheet to your instructor.

Performing CPR—Obstructed Airway on Unconscious Victim	Points Possible	Yes	No	Points Earned	Comments
1. Assembles equipment and supplies and places manikin on firm surface	1				
2. Shakes victim and asks "Are you OK?"	4				
3. If the victim is unconscious, follows "call first, call fast" priorities to call for medical help	4				
4. Opens airway with head-tilt/chin-lift method	4				
5. Looks, listens, and feels for breathing for 5 but not more than 10 seconds	4				
6. Attempts to give breaths	4				
7. When chest does not rise, repositions head and attempts to ventilate	4				
8. Gives abdominal thrusts as follows:					
Positions victim on back	4				
Straddles victim's thighs	4				
Places heel of one hand on abdomen above umbilicus but below xiphoid	4				
Places other hand on top of first hand	4				
Gives quick, upward thrusts into the abdomen	5				
Gives 5 thrusts	5				
9. Checks for object in mouth as follows:					
Opens mouth by lifting lower jaw with thumb and fingers	4				
Uses index finger to sweep mouth with C-shape or hooking motion	4				
Removes object if visible	4				
10. Opens airway and attempts to ventilate	4				
11. If chest rises, continues with steps of CPR by checking carotid pulse	4				
12. If the chest does not rise, repositions head and attempts to ventilate	4				
13. If chest still does not rise, repeats cycle of 5 thrusts, mouth check, attempt to ventilate	4				

212 Copyright © 2004 by Delmar Learning, a division of Thomson Learning, Inc. ALL RIGHTS RESERVED.

Evaluation 13:2E (cont.)

Performing CPR—Obstructed Airway on Unconscious Victim	Points Possible	Yes	No	Points Earned	Comments
14. Continues repeating cycle until object removed and airway open or help comes	4				
15. Follows same sequence for infants but observes following variations:					
Gives 5 back blows by positioning infant face down with head lower than chest	4				
Gives 5 chest thrusts using 2 to 3 fingers one finger's width below an imaginary line drawn between nipples with infant positioned face up and head lower than chest	4				
Looks in mouth for object but sweeps mouth with finger only if object is seen	4				
Attempts to ventilate	4				
16. Cleans and replaces all equipment	1				
Totals	100				

ASSIGNMENT SHEET

Grade _____ Name _____

INTRODUCTION: This assignment will help you review the main facts about providing first aid for bleeding and wounds.

INSTRUCTIONS: Read the information on Providing First Aid for Bleeding and Wounds. In the space provided, print the word(s) that best completes the statement or answers the question.

1. What is the difference between a closed wound and an open wound?

2. First aid care for wounds must be directed at controlling _____ and preventing _____.

3. List the correct name for each of the following types of open wounds.

   a. scrape on the skin:

   b. cut or injury by sharp object:

   c. jagged, irregular injury with tearing:

   d. wound caused by sharp, pointed object:

   e. tissue torn or separated from body:

   f. body part cut off:

4. Briefly describe the characteristics or signs and symptoms for each of the following types of bleeding.

   a. arterial blood:

   b. venous blood:

   c. capillary blood:

5. List the four (4) methods for controlling bleeding in the order in which they should be used.

6. Name two (2) items that can be used to form a protective barrier while controlling bleeding.

7. The main pressure point for the arm is the _____.

   The main pressure point in the leg is the _____.

8. List three (3) ways to prevent infection while caring for minor wounds without severe bleeding.

9. List four (4) signs of infection.

10. If a tetanus infection is a possibility, what first aid is necessary?

11. How should objects embedded deep in the tissues be removed?

12. List four (4) signs and symptoms of a closed wound.

13. List three (3) first aid treatments for a victim of a closed wound.

14. At all times, remain _____ while providing first aid. Obtain _____ care as soon as possible.

PROCEDURE 13:3 PROVIDING FIRST AID FOR BLEEDING AND WOUNDS

Equipment and Supplies

Sterile dressings and bandages, disposable gloves

Procedure

Severe Wounds

1. Follow the steps of priority care, if indicated.
   a. Check the scene. Move the victim only if absolutely necessary.
   b. Check the victim for consciousness and breathing.
   c. Call emergency medical services (EMS).
   d. Provide care to the victim.

2. To control severe bleeding, proceed as follows:
   a. If possible, put on gloves or wrap your hands in plastic wrap to provide a protective barrier while controlling bleeding. If this is not possible in an emergency, use thick layers of dressings and try to avoid contact of blood with your skin.
   b. Using your hand over a thick dressing or sterile gauze, apply pressure directly to the wound.
   c. Continue to apply pressure to the wound for approximately 5 to 10 minutes. Do *not* release the pressure to check whether the bleeding has stopped.
   d. If blood soaks through the first dressing, apply a second dressing on top of the first dressing, and continue to apply direct pressure.
      NOTE: If sterile gauze is *not* available, use clean material or a bare hand.
      CAUTION: Do *not* disturb blood clots once they have formed. Doing so will cause the bleeding to start again.

3. Elevate the injured part above the level of the victim's heart unless a fracture or broken bone is suspected.
   NOTE: This allows gravity to help stop the blood flow to the area.
   NOTE: Direct pressure and elevation are used together. Do *not* stop direct pressure while elevating the part.

4. To hold the dressing in place, apply a pressure bandage. Maintain direct pressure and elevation while applying the pressure bandage. To apply a pressure bandage, proceed as follows:
   a. Apply additional dressings over the dressings already on the wound.
   b. Use a roller bandage to hold the dressings in place by wrapping the roller bandage around the dressings. Use overlapping turns to cover the dressings and to hold them securely in place.
   c. Tie off the ends of the bandage by placing the tie directly over the dressings.
   d. Make sure the pressure bandage is secure. Check a pulse site below the pressure bandage to make sure the bandage is not too tight. A pulse should be present. There should be no discoloration of the skin to indicate poor circulation. If any signs of poor circulation are present, loosen and replace the pressure bandage.

5. If the bleeding continues, it may be necessary to apply pressure to the appropriate pressure point. Continue using direct pressure and elevation and apply pressure to the pressure point as follows:
   a. If the wound is on the arm or hand, apply pressure to the brachial artery. Place the flat surface of your fingers (not your fingertips) against the inside of the victim's upper arm, approximately halfway between the elbow and axilla area. Position your thumb on the outside of the arm. Press your fingers toward your thumb to compress the brachial artery. This decreases the supply of blood to the arm.
   b. If the wound is on the leg, place the flat surfaces of your fingers or the heel of one hand directly over the femoral artery where it passes over the pelvic bone. The position is on the front, middle

part of the upper thigh (groin) where the leg joins the body. Straighten your arm and apply pressure to compress the femoral artery. This decreases the blood supply to the leg.

6. When the bleeding stops, slowly release the pressure on the pressure point. Continue to use direct pressure and elevation. If the bleeding starts again, be ready to reapply pressure to the pressure point.

7. Obtain medical help for the victim as soon as possible. Severe bleeding is a life-threatening emergency.

8. While caring for any victim experiencing severe bleeding, be alert for the signs and symptoms of shock. Treat the victim for shock if any signs or symptoms are noted.

9. During treatment, constantly reassure the victim. Encourage the victim to remain calm by remaining calm yourself.

10. After controlling the bleeding, wash your hands as thoroughly and quickly as possible to avoid contamination from the blood. Wear gloves and use a disinfectant solution to wipe up any blood spills. Always wash your hands thoroughly after removing gloves.

Procedure

Minor Wounds

1. Wash hands thoroughly with soap and water. Put on gloves.

2. Use sterile gauze, soap, and water to wash the wound. Start at the center and wash in an outward direction. Discard the gauze after each pass.

3. Rinse the wound thoroughly with cool water to remove all of the soap.

4. Use sterile gauze to dry the wound. Blot it gently.

5. Apply a sterile dressing to the wound.

6. Caution the victim to look for signs of infection. Tell the victim to obtain medical care if any signs of infection appear.

7. If tetanus infection is possible (for example, in cases involving puncture wounds), tell the victim to contact a doctor regarding a tetanus shot.

   CAUTION: Do *not* use any antiseptic solutions to clean the wound and do *not* apply any substances to the wound unless specifically instructed to do so by your immediate supervisor.

8. Obtain medical help as soon as possible for any victim requiring additional care. Any victim who has particles embedded in a wound, risk of tetanus, severe bleeding, or other complications must be referred for medical care.

9. When care is complete, remove gloves and wash hands thoroughly.

Practice *Use the evaluation sheet for 13:3, Providing First Aid for Bleeding and Wounds, to practice these procedures. When you feel you have mastered these skills, sign the sheet and give it to your instructor for further action.*

✔ **Final Checkpoint** Using the criteria listed on the evaluation sheet, your instructor will grade your performance.

13:3 EVALUATION SHEET

Name _____ Date _____

Evaluated by _____

DIRECTIONS: Practice providing first aid for bleeding and wounds according to the criteria listed. When you are ready for your final check, give this sheet to your instructor.

Providing First Aid for Bleeding and Wounds	Points Possible	Yes	No	Points Earned	Comments
1. Follows priority of care:					
Checks the scene	3				
Checks consciousness and breathing	3				
Calls emergency medical services	3				
Cares for victim	3				
2. Controls severe bleeding with direct pressure:					
Put on gloves or uses protective barrier	3				
Uses dressing over wound	3				
Applies pressure directly to wound	3				
Avoids releasing pressure to check bleeding	3				
Applies second dressing if first soaks through	3				
3. Elevates injured part while applying pressure if no fracture is present	5				
4. Applies pressure bandage to hold dressing in place:					
Maintains direct pressure and elevation	3				
Applies additional dressings over dressings on wound	3				
Secures dressings by wrapping with roller bandage in overlapping turns	3				
Ties off bandage with tie over dressings	3				
Checks pulse site below bandage	3				
Loosens and replaces bandage if signs of poor circulation are present	3				
5. Applies pressure to pressure point if bleeding does not stop:					
Continues with direct pressure and elevation	4				
Applies pressure correctly to brachial artery in arm	4				
Applies pressure correctly to femoral artery in leg	4				
Releases pressure slowly when bleeding stops but continues with direct pressure and elevation	4				

Evaluation 13:3 (cont.)

Providing First Aid for Bleeding and Wounds	Points Possible	Yes	No	Points Earned	Comments
6. Removes gloves and washes hands thoroughly	4				
7. Observes for signs of shock and treats as necessary	4				
8. Reassures victim during care and remains calm	3				
9. Treats minor wounds without severe bleeding:					
Washes hands	2				
Puts on gloves	2				
Washes wound with soap, water, and sterile gauze in outward motion	2				
Discards gauze after each use	2				
Rinses wound with cool water	2				
Blots dry with sterile gauze	2				
Applies sterile dressing	2				
Cautions victim to watch for signs of infection and get medical help	2				
Refers to doctor if danger of tetanus present	2				
Removes gloves and washes hands thoroughly	2				
10. Obtains medical help as soon as possible when needed for victim	3				
Totals	100				

13:4 PROVIDING FIRST AID FOR SHOCK

ASSIGNMENT SHEET

Grade _____ Name _____

INTRODUCTION: This assignment will help you review the main facts regarding shock.

INSTRUCTIONS: Review the information on Providing First Aid for Shock. In the space provided, print the word(s) that best completes the statement or answers the question.

1. Define *shock.*

2. Name the two (2) main body organs affected by an inadequate supply of blood.

3. List four (4) causes of shock.

4. Identify each of the following types of shock:

   a. caused by an acute infection:

   b. heart cannot pump effectively because heart muscle is damaged:

   c. severe bleeding leads to a decrease in blood volume:

   d. hypersensitive or allergic reaction causes body to release histamine:

   e. emotional distress causes sudden dilation of blood vessels:

   f. loss of body fluid causes disruption in normal acid–base balance of body:

5. List six (6) signs or symptoms of shock.

6. The position for treating shock is based on the victim's injuries. Briefly list the best position for each of the following cases:

   a. victim with neck or spine injuries:

   b. victim vomiting or bleeding from the mouth:

   c. victim with respiratory distress:

   d. position if none of the previous conditions is present:

7. A shock victim at an accident scene has been covered with blankets. You notice the victim is perspiring. What should you do?

PROCEDURE 13:4 PROVIDING FIRST AID FOR SHOCK

Equipment and Supplies

Blankets, watch with second hand (optional), disposable gloves

Procedure

1. Follow the steps of priority care, if indicated.
   a. Check the scene. Move the victim only if absolutely necessary.
   b. Check the victim for consciousness and breathing.
   c. Call emergency medical services (EMS).
   d. Provide care to the victim.
   e. Control severe bleeding.
      CAUTION: Follow standard precautions. If possible, wear gloves or use a protective barrier while controlling bleeding.

2. Obtain medical help for the victim as soon as possible. Call or send someone to obtain help.

3. Observe the victim for any signs of shock such as:
   - Look for a pale or bluish color to the skin.
   - Touch the skin and note if it is cool, moist, or clammy to the touch.
   - Note diaphoresis, or excessive perspiration.
   - Check the pulse to see if it is rapid, weak, or irregular. If you are unable to feel a radial pulse, check the carotid pulse.
   - Check the respirations to see if they are rapid, weak, irregular, shallow, or labored.
   - Check blood pressure to see if it is low if equipment is available.
   - Observe the victim for signs of weakness, apathy, or confusion, and check the level of consciousness.
   - Note if the victim is nauseated or vomiting, complaining of excessive thirst, restless or anxious, or complaining of blurred vision.
   - Examine the eyes for a sunken, vacant, or confused appearance, and dilated pupils.

4. Try to reduce the effects or eliminate the cause of shock:
   - Control bleeding by applying pressure at the site.
   - Provide oxygen, if possible.
   - Attempt to ease pain through position changes and comfort measures.
   - Give emotional support.

5. Position the victim based on the injuries or illness present.
   a. If an injury of the neck or spine is present or suspected, do not move the victim.
   b. If the victim has bleeding and injuries to the jaw or mouth or is vomiting, position the victim's body on either side. This allows fluids, vomitus, and/or blood to drain and prevents the airway from becoming blocked by these fluids.
   c. If the victim is having difficulty breathing, position the victim on the back, but raise the head and shoulders slightly to aid breathing.
   d. If the victim has a head injury, position the victim lying flat or with the head raised slightly. **NOTE:** Never allow the head to be positioned lower than the rest of the body.
   e. If none of these conditions exist, position the victim lying flat on the back. To improve circulation, raise the feet and legs 12 inches. If raising the legs causes pain or leads to difficult breathing, however, lower the legs to the flat position.
      CAUTION: Do not raise the legs if the victim has head, neck, or back injuries, or if there are possible fractures of the hips or legs.

Procedure 13:4 (cont.)

    f. If in doubt on how to position a victim according to the injuries involved, keep the victim lying down flat or in the position in which you found him or her. Avoid any unnecessary movement.

6. Place enough blankets or coverings on the victim to prevent chilling. Sometimes, a blanket can be placed between the victim and the ground. Avoid overheating the victim.

7. Do not give the victim anything to eat or drink. If the victim complains of excessive thirst, use a moist cloth to wet the lips, tongue, and inside of the mouth.

8. Constantly reassure the victim. Encourage the victim to remain calm by remaining calm yourself.

9. Observe and provide care to the victim until medical help is obtained.

10. Replace all equipment used. Wash hands.

Practice *Use the evaluation sheet for 13:4, Providing First Aid for Shock, to practice this procedure. When you feel you have mastered this skill, sign the sheet and give it to your instructor for further action.*

✔ **Final Checkpoint** Using the criteria listed on the evaluation sheet, your instructor will grade your performance.

13:4 EVALUATION SHEET

Name _____ Date _____

Evaluated by _____

DIRECTIONS: Practice providing first aid for shock according to the criteria listed. When you are ready for your final check, give this sheet to your instructor.

Providing First Aid for Shock	Points Possible	Yes	No	Points Earned	Comments
1. Follows priorities:					
Checks the scene	4				
Checks consciousness and breathing	4				
Calls emergency medical services	4				
Cares for victim	4				
Controls bleeding	4				
2. Observes victim for signs of shock:					
Pale or bluish color to skin	2				
Cool, moist, or clammy skin	2				
Diaphoresis	2				
Rapid, weak, irregular pulse	2				
Rapid, weak, irregular, shallow, or labored respirations	2				
Low blood pressure	2				
Signs of weakness, apathy, and/or confusion	2				
Nausea and/or vomiting	2				
Excessive thirst	2				
Restlessness or anxiety	2				
Blurred vision	2				
Eyes sunken or vacant, dilated pupils	2				
3. Attempts to reduce shock by treating bleeding, providing oxygen, easing pain, and giving emotional support	6				
4. Positions victim according to injuries or illness:					
Avoids movement if neck or spine injury present	5				
Positions on side if vomiting or has a jaw/mouth injury	5				
Positions lying flat with head raised if victim having difficulty breathing	5				
Positions lying flat or with head raised slightly if head injury present	5				
Positions lying flat with feet raised 12 inches if none of the above conditions present	5				

Providing First Aid for Shock	Points Possible	Yes	No	Points Earned	Comments
5. Places enough blankets on/under victim to prevent chilling but avoids overheating	5				
6. Avoids giving fluids by mouth if medical help is available, victim unconscious or convulsing, brain or abdominal injury, surgery possible, or nausea and vomiting noted	5				
7. Remains calm and reassures victim	5				
8. Observes and cares for victim until medical help obtained	6				
9. Replaces all equipment used	2				
10. Washes hands	2				
Totals	100				

13:5 PROVIDING FIRST AID FOR POISONING

ASSIGNMENT SHEET

Grade _____ Name _____

INTRODUCTION: This assignment will help you review the main facts on providing first aid for poisoning.

INSTRUCTIONS: Read the information on Providing First Aid for Poisoning. In the space provided, print the word(s) that best completes the statement or answers the question.

1. List four (4) ways that poisoning can be caused.

2. What is the first thing to do when a victim swallows a poison?

3. List three (3) types of information that should be given to a poison control center or physician.

4. What should you do if a conscious poisoning victim vomits?

5. How should you position an unconscious poisoning victim who is breathing? Why?

6. List two (2) ways to induce vomiting.

7. Why is activated charcoal used after a poisoning victim vomits?

8. List three (3) types of poisoning victims in whom vomiting should not be induced.

9. What is the first step of treatment for a victim who has been poisoned by inhaling gas?

10. How do you treat victims poisoned by chemicals splashing on the skin?

11. List four (4) signs of an allergic reaction to an injected poison.

Equipment and Supplies

Telephone, disposable gloves

Procedure

1. Follow the steps of priority care, if indicated:
   a. Check the scene. Move the victim only if absolutely necessary.
   b. Check the victim for consciousness and breathing.
   c. Call emergency medical services.
   d. Provide care to the victim.
   e. Control severe bleeding.

   CAUTION: Follow standard precautions. If possible, wear gloves or use a protective barrier while controlling bleeding.

2. Check the victim for signs of poisoning. Signs may include burns on the lips or mouth, odor, a container of poison, or presence of the poisonous substance on the victim or in the victim's mouth. Information may also be obtained from the victim or from an observer.

3. If the victim is *conscious, not convulsing, and has swallowed a poison*:
   a. Try to determine the type of poison, how much was taken, and when the poison was taken. Look for the container near the victim.
   b. Call a poison control center (PCC) or physician immediately for specific information on how to treat the poisoning victim. Provide as much information as possible.
   c. Follow the instructions received from the PCC. Obtain medical help if needed.
   d. If the victim vomits, save a sample of the vomited material.

4. If *the PCC tells you to get the victim to vomit*, induce vomiting. Give the victim warm salt water, or tickle the back of the victim's throat.

   CAUTION: Do *not* induce vomiting if the victim is unconscious or convulsing, has burns on the lips or mouth, or has swallowed an acid, alkali, or petroleum product.

5. If the victim is *unconscious*:
   a. Check for breathing. If the victim is not breathing, give artificial respiration.
   b. If the victim is breathing, position the victim on his or her side to allow fluids to drain from the mouth.
   c. Call a PCC or physician for specific treatment. Obtain medical help immediately.
   d. If possible, save the poison container and a sample of any vomited material. Check with any observers to find out what was taken, how much was taken, and when the poison was taken.

6. If *chemicals or poisons have splashed on the victim's skin*, wash the area thoroughly with large amounts of water. Remove any clothing and jewelry containing the substance. If a large area of the body is affected, a shower, tub, or garden hose may be used to rinse the skin. Obtain medical help immediately for burns or injuries caused by the poison.

7. If the victim has come into *contact with a poisonous plant such as poison ivy, oak, or sumac*, wash the area of contact thoroughly with soap and water. Remove any contaminated clothing. If a rash or weeping sores develop in the next few days after exposure, lotions such as Calamine or Caladryl or a paste made from baking soda and water may help relieve the discomfort. If the condition is severe and affects large areas of the body or face, obtain medical help.

8. If the victim has *inhaled poisonous gas*, do not endanger your life by trying to treat the victim in the area of the gas. Take a deep breath of fresh air before entering the area and hold your breath while you remove the victim from the area. When the victim is in a safe area, check for breathing. Provide artificial respiration, if necessary. Obtain medical help immediately.

Procedure 13:5 (cont.)

9. If poisoning is caused by *injection from an insect bite or sting or a snakebite*, proceed as follows:

   a. If an arm or leg is affected, position the affected area below the level of the heart.

   b. For an *insect bite*, remove any embedded stinger by scraping it off with an object such as a credit card. Wash the area well with soap and water. Apply a sterile dressing and a cold pack to reduce swelling.

   c. If a *tick is embedded* in the skin, use tweezers to gently pull the tick out of the skin. Wash the area thoroughly with soap and water and apply an antiseptic. Obtain medical help if needed.

   d. For a *snakebite*, wash the wound. Immobilize the injured area, positioning it lower than the heart, if possible. Monitor the breathing of the victim and give artificial respiration if necessary. Obtain medical help for the victim as soon as possible.

10. Watch for the signs and symptoms of allergic reaction in all victims. Signs and symptoms of allergic reaction include redness and swelling at the site, itching, hives, pain, swelling of the throat, difficult or labored breathing, dizziness, and a change in the level of consciousness. Maintain respirations and obtain medical help as quickly as possible for the victim experiencing an allergic reaction.

11. Observe for signs of anaphylactic shock while treating any poisoning victim. Treat for shock as necessary.

12. Remain calm while treating the victim. Reassure the victim.

13. Always obtain medical help for any poisoning victim. Some poisons may have delayed reactions. Always keep the telephone numbers of a PCC and other sources of medical assistance in a convenient location so you will be prepared to provide first aid for poisoning.

Practice *Use the evaluation sheet for 13:5, Providing First Aid for Poisoning, to practice this procedure. When you feel you have mastered this skill, sign the sheet and give it to your instructor for further action.*

✔ **Final Checkpoint** Using the criteria listed on the evaluation sheet, your instructor will grade your performance.

13:5 EVALUATION SHEET

Name _____ Date _____

Evaluated by _____

DIRECTIONS: Practice providing first aid for poisoning according to the criteria listed. When you are ready for your final check, give this sheet to your instructor.

Providing First Aid for Poisoning	Points Possible	Yes	No	Points Earned	Comments
1. Follows steps of priority care:					
Checks the scene	2				
Checks consciousness and breathing	2				
Calls emergency medical services	2				
Cares for victim	2				
Controls bleeding	2				
2. Checks victim for signs of poisoning by noting the following points:					
Burns on lips or mouth	2				
Odor	2				
Presence of poison container	2				
Presence of substance on victim or in mouth	2				
Information obtained from victim or observers	2				
3. Provides first aid for conscious victim who has swallowed poison as follows:					
Determines type of poison, how much was taken, and when	2				
Calls poison control center or physician	2				
Follows instructions from poison control center	2				
Saves sample of any vomited material	2				
4. Induces vomiting only if told to do so, no medical help available, and *none* of the following present:					
Victim unconscious	2				
Victim convulsing	2				
Burns on lips or mouth	2				
Victim ingested acid, alkali, or petroleum product	2				
5. Provides first aid for unconscious victim as follows:					
Checks breathing and gives artificial respiration if needed	3				
Positions breathing victim on side	3				
Calls poison control center and obtains medical help	3				

Evaluation 13:5 (cont.)

Providing First Aid for Poisoning	Points Possible	Yes	No	Points Earned	Comments
Saves any vomitus and container with poison	3				
6. Provides first aid for a victim with chemicals or poisons splashed on the skin as follows:					
Washes area with large amounts of water	2				
Removes clothing containing substance	2				
Obtains medical help for burns/injuries	2				
7. Provides first aid for a victim who has come into contact with poisonous plants as follows:					
Washes area with soap and water	2				
Removes contaminated clothing	2				
Applies lotions or baking soda paste	2				
Obtains medical help if condition severe	2				
8. Provides first aid for victim who has inhaled poisonous gas as follows:					
Takes deep breath before entering area	2				
Holds breath while removing victim from area	2				
Checks breathing and gives artificial respiration as needed	2				
Obtains medical help	2				
9. Provides first aid for victim with insect bite/sting or snakebite as follows:					
Positions affected area below level of heart	2				
Treats insect bite/sting:					
Removes embedded stinger by scraping stinger away from skin with the edge of a rigid card	2				
Washes area with soap and water	2				
Applies sterile dressing	2				
Applies cold pack	2				
Treats snakebite:					
Washes wound	2				
Immobilizes injured area	2				
Monitors breathing and gives artificial respiration if necessary	2				
Obtains medical help	2				
Watches for signs/symptoms of allergic reaction	3				
10. Observes all victims for signs of shock and treats as necessary	3				
11. Reassures victim while providing care	3				
12. Obtains medical help for any victim as soon as possible	3				
Totals	100				

13:6 PROVIDING FIRST AID FOR BURNS

ASSIGNMENT SHEET

Grade _____ Name _____

INTRODUCTION: This assignment will help you review the main facts on burns and first aid treatment for burns.

INSTRUCTIONS: Review the information on Providing First Aid for Burns. In the space provided, print the word(s) that best completes the statement or answers the question.

1. Define *burn*.

2. Briefly list the characteristics or signs and symptoms for each of the following types of burn:

   First-degree or   Second-degree or   Third-degree or
   superficial   partial-thickness   full-thickness

3. Identify four (4) situations when medical care should be obtained for burn victims.

4. What is the main treatment for superficial and mild, partial-thickness burns?

5. Why is a sterile dressing applied to a burn?

6. If blisters appear on a burn, how should you treat them?

7. How should severe second-degree or third-degree burns be treated?

8. If chemicals or irritating gases burn the eyes, how should the eyes be treated?

PROCEDURE 13:6 PROVIDING FIRST AID FOR BURNS

Equipment and Supplies

Water, sterile dressings, disposable gloves

Procedure

1. Follow the priorities of care, if indicated:
   a. Check the scene. Move the victim only if absolutely necessary.
   b. Check the victim for consciousness and breathing.
   c. Call emergency medical services (EMS) if necessary.
   d. Provide care to the victim.
   e. Check for bleeding. Control severe bleeding.

   CAUTION: Follow standard precautions. If possible, wear gloves or use a protective barrier while controlling bleeding.

2. Check the burned area carefully to determine the type of burn. A reddened or discolored area is usually a superficial, or first-degree, burn. If the skin is wet, red, swollen, painful, and blistered, the burn is usually a partial-thickness, or second-degree, burn. If the skin is white or charred and there is destruction of tissue, the burn is a full-thickness, or third-degree, burn.

   NOTE: Victims can have more than one type of burn at the same time. Treat for the most severe type of burn present.

3. For a *first-degree or mild second-degree burn:*
   a. Cool the burn by flushing it with large amounts of cool water. If this is not possible, apply clean or sterile cloths that are cold and wet. Continue applying cold water until the pain subsides.
   b. Use sterile gauze to gently blot the injured area dry.
   c. Apply dry, sterile dressings to the burned area. If possible, use nonadhesive (nonstick) dressings, because they will not stick to the burn.
   d. If blisters are present, do *not* break or open them.
   e. If possible, elevate the burned area to reduce swelling caused by inflammation.
   f. Obtain medical help for burns to the face, or if burns cover more than 15 percent of the surface of an adult's body or 10 percent of the surface of a child's body. If the victim is having difficulty breathing, or any other distress is noted, obtain medical help.
   g. Do *not* apply any cotton, ointment, powders, grease, butter, or similar substances to the burned area.
      NOTE: These substances may increase the possibility of infection.

4. For a *severe second-degree or any third-degree burn:*
   a. Call for medical help immediately.
   b. Use thick, sterile dressings to cover the injured areas.
   c. Do *not* attempt to remove any particles of clothing that have stuck to the burned areas.
   d. If the hands and arms or legs and feet are affected, elevate these areas.
   e. If the victim has burns on the face or is experiencing difficulty in breathing, elevate the head.
   f. Watch the victim closely for signs of shock and provide care if necessary.

5. For a *burn caused by a chemical splashing on the skin:*
   a. Using large amounts of cool water, immediately flush the area for 15 to 30 minutes or until medical help arrives.
   b. Remove any articles of clothing, socks and shoes, or jewelry contaminated by the substance.
   c. Continue flushing the area with large amounts of cool water.
   d. Obtain medical help immediately.

Procedure 13:6 (cont.)

6. If the *eye has been burned by chemicals or irritating gases:*

   a. If the victim is wearing contact lenses or glasses, ask him or her to remove them quickly.

   b. Tilt the victim's head toward the injured side.

   c. Hold the eyelid of the injured eye open. Pour cool water from the inner part of the eye (the part closest to the nose) toward the outer part.

   d. Use cool water to irrigate the eye for 15 to 30 minutes or until medical help arrives.
      CAUTION: Take care that the water or chemicals do not enter the uninjured eye.

   e. Obtain medical help immediately.

7. Observe for signs of shock in all burn victims. Treat for shock as necessary.

8. Reassure the victim as you are providing treatment. Remain calm and encourage the victim to remain calm.

9. Obtain medical help immediately for any burn victim with extensive burns, third-degree burns, burns to the face, signs of shock, respiratory distress, eye burns, and/or chemical burns to the skin.

Practice *Use the evaluation sheet for 13:6, Providing First Aid for Burns, to practice this procedure. When you feel you have mastered this skill, sign the sheet and give it to your instructor for further action.*

✔ **Final Checkpoint** Using the criteria listed on the evaluation sheet, your instructor will grade your performance.

Name _____ Date _____

Evaluated by _____

DIRECTIONS: Practice providing first aid for burns according to the criteria listed. When you are ready for your final check, give this sheet to your instructor.

Providing First Aid for Burns	Points Possible	Yes	No	Points Earned	Comments
1. Follows priorities:					
Checks the scene	2				
Checks consciousness and breathing	2				
Calls emergency medical services	2				
Cares for victim	2				
Controls bleeding	2				
2. Identifies type of burn present as follows:					
First-degree or superficial: reddened	3				
Second-degree or partial-thickness: red, wet, painful, swollen, blistered	3				
Third-degree or full-thickness: white or charred with destruction of tissue	3				
3. Provides first aid for superficial or mild partial-thickness burns as follows:					
Cools burn by flushing it with large amounts of cool water	3				
Blots dry gently with sterile gauze	3				
Applies dry sterile dressing	3				
Avoids breaking blisters	3				
Elevates burned area if possible	3				
Obtains medical help if necessary	3				
4. Provides first aid for severe partial-thickness and all full-thickness burns as follows:					
Obtains medical help immediately	3				
Applies dry, sterile dressing	3				
Avoids removing charred clothing from area	3				
Elevates hands and arms or legs and feet if affected	3				
Elevates head if victim in respiratory distress	3				
5. Provides first aid for chemical burns as follows:					
Flushes area with large amounts of cool water	3				
Removed contaminated clothing	3				
Continues flushing with large amounts of cool water	3				
Obtains medical help	3				

Evaluation 13:6 (cont.)

Providing First Aid for Burns	Points Possible	Yes	No	Points Earned	Comments
6. Provides first aid for burns of the eye as follows:					
Asks victim to remove glasses or contacts	2				
Positions victim with head to side and injured eye down	3				
Pours water from inner to outer part of eye	3				
Irrigates for 15–30 minutes or until medical help arrives	3				
Obtains medical help	3				
7. Observes for signs of shock in all victims and treats as necessary	3				
8. Reassures victim and remains calm	3				
9. Obtains medical help for any of the following:					
Burns extensive (over 15% of surface of adult body, 10% in child)	2				
Third-degree or full-thickness burns	2				
Victim under 5 or over 60 with partial-thickness burn	2				
Burns of the face	2				
Signs of shock	2				
Respiratory distress	2				
Burns of the eye/eyes	2				
Chemical burns on the skin	2				
Totals	100				

ASSIGNMENT SHEET

Grade _____ Name _____

INTRODUCTION: This assignment will help you review the main facts regarding conditions caused by exposure to heat.

INSTRUCTIONS: Review the information on Providing First Aid for Heat Exposure. In the space provided, print the word(s) that best completes the statement or answers the question.

1. What occurs when the body is overexposed to heat?

2. What are heat cramps?

3. List two (2) first aid treatments for heat cramps.

4. List four (4) signs or symptoms of heat exhaustion.

5. List two (2) first aid treatments for heat exhaustion.

6. How does internal body temperature differ in heat exhaustion and heat stroke?

7. List three (3) signs and symptoms of heat stroke.

8. High body temperatures (such as 105° F or 41°C) can cause _____ and/or _____ in a very short period of time.

9. List two (2) first aid treatments for heat stroke.

10. Identify two (2) precautions a victim should take after recovering from any condition caused by exposure to heat.

Equipment and Supplies

Water, wash cloths or small towels

Procedure

1. Follow the priorities of care, if indicated:
   a. Check the scene. Move the victim only if absolutely necessary.
   b. Check the victim for consciousness and breathing.
   c. Call emergency medical services (EMS) if necessary.
   d. Provide care to the victim.
   e. Check for bleeding. Control severe bleeding.
      CAUTION: Follow standard precautions. If possible, wear gloves or use a protective barrier while controlling bleeding.

2. Observe the victim closely for signs and symptoms of heat exposure. Information may also be obtained directly from the victim or from observers.
   a. If the victim has been exposed to heat or has been exercising strenuously and is complaining of muscular pain or spasm, he or she is probably experiencing heat cramps.
   b. If the victim has close-to-normal body temperature but has pale and clammy skin, is perspiring excessively, and complains of nausea, headache, weakness, dizziness, or fatigue, he or she is probably experiencing heat exhaustion.
   c. If body temperature is high (105°F, or 40.6°C, or higher); skin is red, dry, and hot; and the victim is weak or unconscious, he or she is experiencing heat stroke.

3. If the victim has *heat cramps*:
   a. Use your hand to apply firm pressure to the cramped muscle(s). This helps relieve the spasms.
   b. Encourage relaxation. Allow the victim to lie down in a cool area, if possible.
   c. If the victim is alert and conscious and is not nauseated or vomiting, give him or her small sips of cool water, approximately 4 ounces every 15 minutes.
   d. If the heat cramps continue or get worse, obtain medical help.

4. If the victim has *heat exhaustion*:
   a. Move the victim to a cool area, if possible. An air-conditioned room is ideal, but a fan can also help circulate air and cool the victim.
   b. Help the victim lie down flat on the back. Elevate the victim's feet and legs 12 inches.
   c. Loosen any tight clothing. Remove excessive clothing such as jackets and sweaters.
   d. Apply cool, wet cloths to the victim's face.
   e. If the victim is conscious and is not nauseated or vomiting, give him or her small sips of cool water, approximately 4 ounces every 15 minutes.
   f. If the victim complains of nausea and/or vomits, discontinue water. Obtain medical help.

5. If the victim has *heat stroke*:
   a. Immediately move the victim to a cool area, if possible.
   b. Remove excessive clothing.
   c. Sponge the bare skin with cool water, or place ice or cold packs on the victim's wrists, ankles, and in the axillary and groin areas. The victim can also be placed in a tub of cool water to lower body temperature.
      CAUTION: Watch that the victim's head is not submerged in water. If the victim is unconscious, you may need assistance to place him or her in the tub.
   d. If vomiting occurs, position the victim on his or her side.

Procedure 13:7 (cont.)

    e. Watch for signs of difficulty in breathing and provide care as indicated.

    f. Obtain medical help immediately. This is a life-threatening emergency.

6. Shock can develop quickly in all victims of heat exposure. Be alert for the signs of shock and treat as necessary.

    CAUTION: Obtain medical help for heat cramps that do not subside, heat exhaustion with signs of shock or vomiting, and *all* heat stroke victims as soon as possible.

7. Reassure the victim as you are providing treatment. Remain calm.

Practice *Use the evaluation sheet for 13:7, Providing First Aid for Heat Exposure, to practice this procedure. When you feel you have mastered this skill, sign the sheet and give it to your instructor for further action.*

✔ **Final Checkpoint** Using the criteria listed on the evaluation sheet, your instructor will grade your performance.

13:7 EVALUATION SHEET

Name _____ Date _____

Evaluated by _____

DIRECTIONS: Practice providing first aid for heat exposure according to the criteria listed. When you are ready for your final check, give this sheet to your instructor.

Providing First Aid for Heat Exposure	Points Possible	Yes	No	Points Earned	Comments
1. Follows priorities:					
Checks the scene	2				
Checks consciousness and breathing	2				
Calls emergency medical services	2				
Cares for victim	2				
Controls bleeding	2				
2. Observes signs to determine condition as follows:					
Heat cramps: muscle pain or spasm	3				
Heat exhaustion: close to normal body temperature, skin pale and clammy, diaphoresis, nausea, headache, weakness, dizziness, fatigue	4				
Heat stroke: high body temperature; skin hot, red, and dry; weak or unconscious	4				
3. Provides first aid for heat cramps as follows:					
Applies firm pressure to muscle with hand	4				
Lays victim down in cool area	4				
Gives victim small sips of cool water to total 4 ounces in 15 minutes	4				
Obtains medical help if cramps continue	4				
4. Provides first aid for heat exhaustion as follows:					
Moves victim to cool area	3				
Positions victim lying down with feet elevated 12 inches	3				
Loosens tight clothing from victim	3				
Applies cool, wet cloths	3				
Gives victim small sips of cool water to total 4 ounces in 15 minutes	3				
Discontinues water if victim complains of nausea and/or vomits	3				
Obtains medical help if necessary	3				

Name _____

Evaluation 13:7 (cont.)

Providing First Aid for Heat Exposure	Points Possible	Yes	No	Points Earned	Comments
5. Provides first aid for heat stroke as follows:					
Moves victim to cool area	4				
Removes excess clothing from victim	4				
Sponges skin with cool water; places ice or cold packs on victim's wrists, angles, and in axillary or groin areas; or puts victim in tub of cool water	4				
Positions victim on side if vomiting occurs	4				
Obtains medical help immediately	4				
6. Observes for signs of shock and treats for shock in all victims	5				
7. Reassures victim while providing care, remains calm	5				
8. Obtains medical help for any of the following victims:					
Heat cramps that do not subside	4				
Heat exhaustion victim with vomiting or shock	4				
All heat stroke victims	4				
Totals	100				

13:8 PROVIDING FIRST AID FOR COLD EXPOSURE

ASSIGNMENT SHEET

Grade _____ Name _____

INTRODUCTION: This assignment will help you review the main facts on first aid for cold exposure.

INSTRUCTIONS: Read the information on Providing First Aid for Cold Exposure. In the space provided, print the word(s) that best completes the statement or answers the question.

1. List two (2) factors that affect the degree of injury caused by exposure to the cold.

2. List four (4) symptoms that can result from prolonged exposure to the cold.

3. List two (2) first aid treatments for hypothermia.

4. What is frostbite?

5. List three (3) symptoms of frostbite.

6. Name three (3) common sites for frostbite.

7. What temperature water should be used to warm a body part injured by frostbite?

8. Why is it important not to rub or massage a body part affected by frostbite?

9. How should you treat blisters that form on frost-damaged skin?

10. Why do you place sterile gauze between fingers or toes that have been injured by frostbite?

Equipment and Supplies

Blankets, bath water and thermometer, sterile gauze sponges

Procedure

1. Follow the priorities of care, if indicated:
   a. Check the scene. Move the victim only if absolutely necessary.
   b. Check the victim for consciousness and breathing.
   c. Call emergency medical services (EMS) if necessary.
   d. Provide care to the victim.
   e. Check for bleeding. Control severe bleeding.
      CAUTION: Follow standard precautions. If possible, wear gloves or use a protective barrier while controlling bleeding.

2. Observe the victim closely for signs and symptoms of cold exposure. Information may also be obtained directly from the victim or observers. Note shivering, numbness, weakness or drowsiness, confusion, low body temperature, and lethargy. Check the skin, particularly on the toes, fingers, ears, nose, and cheeks. Suspect frostbite if any areas are pale, glossy, white or grayish-yellow, and cold to the touch, and if the victim complains of any part of the body feeling numb or painless.

3. Move the victim to a warm area as soon as possible.

4. Immediately remove any wet or frozen clothing. Loosen any tight clothing that decreases circulation.

5. Slowly warm the victim by wrapping the victim in blankets or dressing the victim in dry, warm clothing.
   CAUTION: Warm a victim of hypothermia slowly. Rapid warming can cause heart problems or increase circulation to the surface of the body, which causes additional cooling of vital organs.

6. If a body part is affected by frostbite, immerse the part in warm water measuring 100°F to 104°F (37.8°C to 40°C).
   CAUTION: Do *not* use heat lamps, hot water above the stated temperatures, or heat from stoves or ovens. Excessive heat can burn the victim.

7. After the body part affected by frostbite has been thawed and the skin becomes flushed, discontinue warming the area because swelling may develop rapidly. Dry the part by blotting gently with a towel or soft cloth. Gently wrap the part in clean or sterile cloths. Use sterile gauze to separate the fingers and/or toes to prevent them from rubbing together.
   CAUTION: *Never* rub or massage the frostbitten area, because doing so can cause gangrene.

8. Help the victim lie down. Do not allow the victim to walk or stand if the legs, feet, or toes are injured. Elevate any injured areas.

9. Observe the victim for signs of shock. Treat for shock as necessary.

10. If the victim is conscious and is not nauseated or vomiting, give warm liquids to drink.
    CAUTION: Do *not* give beverages containing alcohol or caffeine. Give the victim warm broth, water, or milk.

11. Reassure the victim while providing treatment. Remain calm and encourage the victim to remain calm.

12. Obtain medical help as soon as possible.

Practice *Use the evaluation sheet for 13:8, Providing First Aid for Cold Exposure, to practice this procedure. When you feel you have mastered this skill, sign the sheet and give it to your instructor for further action.*

✔ **Final Checkpoint** Using the criteria listed on the evaluation sheet, your instructor will grade your performance.

Name _____ Date _____

Evaluated by _____

DIRECTIONS: Practice providing first aid for cold exposure according to the criteria listed. When you are ready for your final check, give this sheet to your instructor.

Providing First Aid for Cold Exposure	Points Possible	Yes	No	Points Earned	Comments
1. Follows priorities:					
Checks the scene	3				
Checks consciousness and breathing	3				
Calls emergency medical services	3				
Cares for victim	3				
Controls severe bleeding	3				
2. Observes for signs of exposure to cold	7				
3. Checks skin for signs of frostbite	6				
4. Moves victim to warm area	6				
5. Removes wet or frozen clothing and loosens constrictive clothing	6				
6. Warms victim slowly by wrapping in blankets or putting on dry clothing	6				
7. Immerses frostbitten part in water at 100°–104°F (37.8–40°C)	6				
8. Discontinues warming when skin flushed	6				
9. Dries area of body by blotting gently	6				
10. Places sterile gauze between fingers and toes affected by frostbite	6				
11. Positions victim lying down with affected parts elevated	6				
12. Observes and treats for shock	6				
13. Gives warm liquids to victim if victim conscious and not nauseated or vomiting	6				
14. Reassures victim while providing care	6				
15. Obtains medical help as soon as possible	6				
Totals	100				

ASSIGNMENT SHEET

Grade ——————————————— Name ———————————————————————————

INTRODUCTION: This assignment will help you review the main facts regarding bone and joint injuries.

INSTRUCTIONS: Read the information on Providing First Aid for Bone and Joint Injuries. In the space provided, print the word(s) that best completes the statement or answers the question.

1. Define each of the following:

   fracture:

   dislocation:

   sprain:

   strain:

2. What is the difference between a closed or simple fracture and an open or compound fracture?

3. List four (4) signs and symptoms of a fracture.

4. List three (3) signs and symptoms of a dislocation.

5. Why is movement of the injured part dangerous when a dislocation has occurred?

6. List three (3) signs and symptoms of a sprain.

7. List two (2) first aid treatments for a sprain.

8. Why are cold applications used to treat a sprain or strain?

9. Why are warm applications used to treat a strain?

10. List four (4) different types of materials that can be used for splints.

11. List three (3) basic principles that should be followed when splints are applied.

12. How can you test that an air splint is inflated properly?

13. Why should the hand be positioned higher than the elbow when a sling is applied?

14. List four (4) points you can check to make sure that circulation is not impaired after a splint or sling has been applied.

15. What should you do if you notice signs of impaired circulation after applying a splint?

16. Why is it best to avoid moving any victim who has a neck or spine injury?

PROCEDURE 13:9 PROVIDING FIRST AID FOR BONE AND JOINT INJURIES

Equipment and Supplies

Blankets, splints of various sizes, air or inflatable splints, triangular bandages, strips of cloth or roller gauze, disposable gloves

Procedure

1. Follow the priorities of care, if indicated:

   a. Check the scene. Move the victim only if absolutely necessary. If the victim must be moved from a dangerous area, pull in the direction of the long axis of the body (that is, from the head or feet). If at all possible, tie an injured leg to the other leg or secure an injured arm to the body before movement.
   CAUTION: If neck or spine injuries are suspected, avoid any movement of the victim unless movement is necessary to save the victim's life.

   b. Check the victim for consciousness and breathing.

   c. Call emergency medical services (EMS) if necessary.

   d. Provide care to the victim.

   e. Control severe bleeding. If an open wound accompanies a fracture, take care not to push broken bone ends into the wound.
    CAUTION: Follow standard precautions. If possible, wear gloves or use a protective barrier while controlling bleeding.

2. Observe for signs and symptoms of a fracture, dislocation, or joint injury. Note deformities (such as a shortening or lengthening of an extremity), limited motion or loss of motion, pain, tenderness, swelling, discoloration, and bone fragments protruding through the skin. Also, the victim may state that he or she heard a bone snap or crack, or may complain of a grating sensation.

3. Immobilize the injured part to prevent movement.

   CAUTION: Do *not* attempt to straighten a deformity, replace broken bone ends, or reduce a dislocation. Avoid any unnecessary movement of the injured part. If a bone injury is suspected, treat the victim as though a fracture or dislocation has occurred. Use splints or slings to immobilize the injured part.

4. *To apply splints:*

   a. Obtain commercial splints or improvise splints by using blankets, pillows, newspapers, boards, cardboard, or similar supportive materials.

   b. Make sure that the splints are long enough to immobilize the joint both above and below the injury.

   c. Position the splints, making sure that they do *not* apply pressure directly at the site of injury. Two splints are usually used. However, if a pillow, blanket, or similar item is used, one such item can be rolled around the area to provide support on all sides.

   d. Use thick dressings, cloths, towels, or other similar materials to pad the splints. Make sure bony areas are protected. Avoid direct contact between the splint material and the skin.
   NOTE: Many commercial splints are already padded. However, additional padding is often needed to protect the bony areas.

   e. Use strips of cloth, triangular bandages folded into strips, roller gauze, or other similar material to tie or anchor the splints in place. The use of elastic bandages is discouraged because the bandages may cut off or interfere with circulation. If splints are long, three to five ties may be required. Tie the strips above and below the upper joint and above and below the lower joint. An additional tie should be placed in the center region of the splint.

   f. Avoid any unnecessary movement of the injured area while splints are being applied. If possible, have another individual support the area while you are applying the splints.

Procedure 13:9 (cont.)

5. *To apply air (inflatable) splints:*
   a. Obtain the correct splint for the injured part.
      NOTE: Most air splints are available for full arm, lower arm, wrist, full leg, lower leg, and ankle/foot.
   b. Some air splints have zippers for easier application, but others must be slipped into position on the victim. If the splint has a zipper, position the open splint on the injured area, taking care to avoid any movement of the affected part. Use your hand to support the injured area. Close the zipper. If the splint must be slipped into position, slide the splint onto your arm first. Then hold the injured leg or arm and slide the splint from your arm to the victim's injured extremity. This technique prevents unnecessary movement.
   c. Inflate the splint. Many splints are inflated by blowing into the nozzle. Others require the use of a pressure solution in a can. Follow instructions provided by the manufacturer of the splint.
   d. Check to make sure that the splint is not overinflated. Use your thumb to press a section of the splint. Your thumb should leave a slight indentation if the splint is inflated correctly.

6. *To apply a sling,* follow the manufacturer's instructions for commercial slings. To use a triangular bandage for a sling, proceed as follows:
   a. If possible, obtain the help of another individual to support the injured arm while the sling is being applied. Sometimes, the victim can hold the injured arm in place.
   b. Place the long straight edge of the triangular bandage on the uninjured side. Allow one end to extend over the shoulder of the uninjured arm. The other end should hang down in front of the victim's chest. The short edge of the triangle should extend back and under the elbow of the injured arm.
      CAUTION: Avoid excessive movement of the injured limb while positioning the sling.
   c. Bring the long end of the bandage up and over the shoulder of the injured arm.
   d. Use a square knot to tie the two ends together near the neck. Make sure the knot is not over a bone. Tie it to either side of the spinal column. Place gauze or padding between the knot and the skin.
   e. Adjust the sling to make sure the hand is elevated 5 to 6 inches above the elbow.
   f. The point of the bandage is now near the elbow. Bring the point forward, fold it, and pin it to the front of the sling. If no pin is available, coil the end and tie it in a knot.
      CAUTION: If you use a pin, put your hand between the pin and the victim's skin while inserting the pin.
   g. Check the position of the sling. The fingers of the injured hand should extend beyond the edge of the triangular bandage. In addition, the hand should be slightly elevated to prevent swelling (edema).

7. After splints and/or slings have been applied, check for signs of impaired circulation, such as:
   - Skin color should be pink. A pale or bluish color is a sign of poor circulation.
   - Skin should be warm to the touch.
   - Swelling can indicate poor circulation.
   - The victim complains of pain or pressure from the splints and/or slings, or of numbness or tingling in the area below the splints/sling.
   - Slightly press the nail beds on the foot or hand so they temporarily turn white. If circulation is good, the pink color will return to the nail beds immediately after pressure is released.

   If you note any signs of impaired circulation, loosen the splints and/or sling immediately.

8. Watch for signs of shock in any victim with a bone and/or joint injury. Remember, inadequate blood flow is the main cause of shock. Watch for signs of impaired circulation, such as a bluish tinge around the lips or nail beds. Treat for shock, as necessary.

9. If medical help is delayed, cold applications such as cold compresses or an ice bag can be used on the injured area to decrease swelling.
   CAUTION: To prevent injury to the skin, make sure that the ice bag is covered with a towel or other material.

Procedure 13:9 (cont.)

10. Place the victim in a comfortable position, but avoid any unnecessary movement.

    CAUTION: Avoid *any* movement if a neck or spine injury is suspected.

11. Reassure the victim while providing first aid. Try to relieve the pain by carefully positioning the injured part, avoiding unnecessary movement, and applying cold.

12. Obtain medical help as quickly as possible.

Practice *Use the evaluation sheet for 13:9, Providing First Aid for Bone and Joint Injuries, to practice this procedure. When you feel you have mastered this skill, sign the sheet and give it to your instructor for further action.*

✔ **Final Checkpoint** Using the criteria listed on the evaluation sheet, your instructor will grade your performance.

Name _____ Date _____

Evaluated by _____

DIRECTIONS: Practice providing first aid for bone and joint injuries according to the criteria listed. When you are ready for your final check, give this sheet to your instructor.

Providing First Aid for Bone and Joint Injuries	Points Possible	Yes	No	Points Earned	Comments
1. Follows priorities of care:					
Checks the scene	2				
Checks consciousness and breathing	2				
Calls emergency medical services	2				
Cares for victim	2				
Controls bleeding	2				
2. Observes victim for signs of bone or joint injury	3				
3. Immobilizes any injured area or suspected fracture and/or dislocation	3				
4. Applies splints:					
Selects appropriate splint material	3				
Uses splints that will immobilize joint above and below injured area	3				
Positions splints correctly to avoid pressure on injury	3				
Pads splints especially at bony areas	3				
Ties splints in place	3				
Avoids any unnecessary movement during application	3				
5. Applies air/inflatable splints as follows:					
Obtains correct splint	3				
Supports injured area while positioning splint	3				
Inflates splint correctly	3				
Checks inflation by pressing on splint with thumb	3				
6. Applies sling with triangular bandage:					
Provides support for arm while applying	3				
Positions bandage with long edge on uninjured side	3				
Brings lower end up over injured arm and over shoulder on injured side	3				
Ties bandage ends with square knot avoiding bony area of neck and places padding between knot and skin	3				

Evaluation 13:9 (cont.)

Providing First Aid for Bone and Joint Injuries	Points Possible	Yes	No	Points Earned	Comments
Secures area by elbow with pin or by tying in knot	3				
Checks to be sure fingers are exposed and hand is elevated 5 to 6 inches above elbow	3				
7. Checks for signs of impaired circulation by noting the following:					
Pale or bluish color	2				
Cold to touch	2				
Swelling/edema	2				
Pain or pressure from splint/sling	2				
Numbness or tingling	2				
Poor return of pink color after blanching nails	2				
8. Loosens splint/sling if impaired circulation noted	4				
9. Observes for signs of shock and treats as needed	4				
10. Applies cold applications to reduce swelling and pain	4				
11. Positions victim in a comfortable position but avoids unnecessary movement and avoids all movement if neck or spine injury suspected	4				
12. Reassures victim while providing first aid care	4				
13. Obtains medical help as soon as possible	4				
Totals	100				

13:10 PROVIDING FIRST AID FOR SPECIFIC INJURIES

ASSIGNMENT SHEET

Grade _____ Name _____

INTRODUCTION: This assignment will help you review the specific care given to victims with injuries to the eye, ear, nose, brain, chest, abdomen, and genital organs.

INSTRUCTIONS: Read the information on Providing First Aid for Specific Injuries. In the space provided, print the word(s) that best completes the statement or answers the question.

1. Injuries to the eye always involve the danger of _____. A top priority of first aid care is to obtain the assistance of _____, preferably a/an _____.

2. Briefly describe two (2) techniques that can be used to remove a foreign object that is floating free in the eye.

3. If an object is embedded in the eye, what first aid care should be given?

4. List the steps of first aid treatment that should be followed when an object is protruding from the eye.

5. How should you care for tissue torn from the ear?

6. How should you position a victim with cerebrospinal fluid draining from the ear?

7. List four (4) signs and symptoms of injuries to the brain.

8. List three (3) aspects of first aid care for victims with brain injuries.

9. List two (2) causes of an epistaxis or nosebleed.

10. How should you position a victim with a nosebleed?

11. What type of dressing should be applied to a sucking chest wound? Why?

12. How should you position a victim with a sucking chest wound?

13. List three (3) signs and symptoms of abdominal injury.

14. How should you position a victim with an abdominal injury?

15. How should you care for abdominal organs protruding from a wound?

Equipment and Supplies

Blankets, pillows, dressings, bandages, tape, aluminum foil or plastic wrap, eye shields or sterile dressings, sterile water, disposable gloves

Procedure

1. Follow the priorities of care, if indicated:
   a. Check the scene. Move the victim only if absolutely necessary.
   b. Check the victim for consciousness and breathing.
   c. Call emergency medical services (EMS), if necessary.
   d. Provide care to the victim.
   e. Check for bleeding. Control severe bleeding.
      CAUTION: Follow standard precautions. If possible, wear gloves or use a protective barrier while controlling bleeding.

2. Observe the victim closely for signs and symptoms of specific injuries. Do a systematic examination of the victim. Always have a reason for everything you do. Explain what you are doing to the victim and/or observers.

3. *If the victim has an eye injury*, proceed as follows:
   a. If the victim has a *free-floating particle or foreign body in the eye*, warn the victim *not* to rub the eye. Wash your hands thoroughly to prevent infection. Gently grasp the upper eyelid and draw it down over the lower eyelid. If this does not remove the object, use your thumb and forefinger to grasp the eyelashes and gently raise the upper eyelid. Tell the victim to look down and tilt his or her head slightly to the injured side. Use water to gently flush the eye or use the corner of a piece of sterile gauze to gently remove the object. If this does not remove the object or if the object is embedded, proceed to step b.
   b. If an *object is embedded in the eye*, make *no* attempt to remove it. Rather, apply a dry, sterile dressing to loosely cover the eye. Obtain medical help.
   c. If an eye injury has caused a *contusion, a black eye, internal bleeding, and/or torn tissue in the eye*, apply sterile dressings or eye shields to both eyes. Keep the victim lying flat. Obtain medical help. **NOTE:** Both eyes are covered to prevent involuntary movement of the injured eye.
   d. If an *object is protruding from the eye*, make *no* attempt to remove the object. If possible, support the object in position by loosely placing dressings around it. A paper cup with the bottom removed can also be used to surround and prevent any movement of the object. Apply dressings to the uninjured eye to prevent movement of the injured eye. Keep the victim lying flat. Obtain medical help immediately.

4. *If the victim has an ear injury:*
   a. Control severe bleeding from an ear wound by using a sterile dressing to apply light pressure.
      CAUTION: Follow standard precautions. Wear gloves or use a protective barrier to prevent contamination from the blood.
   b. If any *tissue has been torn from the ear*, preserve the tissue by placing it in cool, sterile water or normal saline solution. The tissue may also be put in sterile gauze that has been moistened with sterile water. Send the torn tissue to the medical facility along with the victim. **NOTE:** If sterile water is not available, use cool, clean water.
   c. If a *rupture or perforation of the eardrum* is suspected or evident, place sterile gauze loosely in the outer ear canal. Caution the victim against hitting the side of the head to restore hearing. Obtain medical help.
   d. If *cerebrospinal fluid is draining from the ear*, make no attempt to stop the flow of the fluid. If no neck or spine injury is suspected, turn the victim on his or her injured side and slightly elevate the

head and shoulders to allow the fluid to drain. A dressing may be positioned to absorb the flow. Obtain medical help immediately.

CAUTION: Follow standard precautions. Wear gloves or use a protective barrier to prevent contamination from the cerebrospinal fluid.

5. *If the victim has a brain injury:*

   a. Keep the victim lying flat. Treat for shock. If there is no evidence of a neck or spine injury, place a small pillow or a rolled blanket or coat under the victim's head and shoulders to elevate the head slightly.

   CAUTION: Never position the victim's head lower than the rest of the body.

   b. Watch closely for signs of respiratory distress. Provide artificial respiration if needed.
   NOTE: Remove the pillow if artificial respiration is given.

   c. If cerebrospinal fluid is draining from the ears, nose, and/or mouth, make *no* attempt to stop the flow. Position dressings to absorb the flow.

   CAUTION: Follow standard precautions. Wear gloves or use a protective barrier to prevent contamination from the cerebrospinal fluid.

   d. Avoid giving the victim any fluids by mouth. If the victim complains of excessive thirst, use a cool, wet cloth to moisten the lips, tongue, and inside of the mouth.

   e. If the victim is unconscious, note for how long and report this information to the emergency rescue personnel.

   f. Obtain medical help as quickly as possible.

6. *If the victim has a nosebleed:*

   a. Try to keep the victim calm. Remain calm yourself.

   b. Position the victim in a sitting position, if possible. Lean the head forward slightly. If the victim cannot sit up, slightly elevate the head.

   c. Apply pressure by pressing the nostril(s) toward the midline. Continue applying pressure for at least 5 minutes and longer if necessary to control the bleeding.
   NOTE: If both nostrils are bleeding and must be pressed toward the midline, tell the victim to breathe through the mouth.

   CAUTION: Follow standard precautions. Wear gloves or use a protective barrier to prevent contamination from the blood.

   d. If application of pressure does not control the bleeding, insert gauze into the bleeding nostril, taking care to allow some of the gauze to hang out. Then apply pressure again by pushing the nostril toward the midline.

   e. Apply cold compresses to the bridge of the nose. Use cold, wet cloths or a covered ice bag.

   f. If the bleeding does not stop, a fracture is suspected, or the victim has repeated nosebleeds, obtain medical help.
   NOTE: Nosebleeds can indicate a serious underlying condition that requires medical attention, such as high blood pressure.

7. *If the victim has a chest injury:*

   a. If the wound is a sucking chest wound, apply a nonporous dressing. Use plastic wrap or aluminum foil to create an airtight seal. Use tape on three sides to hold the dressing in place. Leave the fourth side loose to allow excess air to escape when the victim exhales.

   b. Maintain an open airway. Constantly be alert for signs of respiratory distress. Provide artificial respiration as needed.

   c. If there is no evidence of a neck or spine injury, position the victim with his or her injured side down. Slightly elevate the head and chest by placing small pillows or blankets under the victim.

   d. If an object is protruding from the chest, make *no* attempt to remove it. If possible, immobilize the object with dressings, and tape around it.

   e. Obtain medical help immediately for all chest injuries.

8. *If the victim has an abdominal injury:*

   a. Position the victim flat on the back. Place a small pillow or a rolled blanket or coat under the victim's knees to flex (bend) them slightly. Elevate the head and shoulders to aid breathing. If movement of the legs causes pain, leave the victim lying flat.

   b. If abdominal organs are protruding from the wound, make *no* attempt to reposition the organs. Remove clothing from around the wound or protruding organs. Use a sterile dressing that has been moistened with sterile water or normal saline solution to cover the area. If sterile water or normal saline is not available, use warm tap water to moisten the dressings.

   c. Cover the dressing with plastic wrap, if available, to keep the dressing moist. Then apply a folded towel or aluminum foil to keep the area warm.

   d. Avoid giving the victim any fluids or food. If the victim complains of excessive thirst, use a cool, wet cloth to moisten the lips, tongue, and inside of the mouth.

   e. Obtain medical help immediately.

9. *If the victim has an injury to the genital organs:*

   a. Control severe bleeding by using a sterile dressing to apply direct pressure.
      CAUTION: Follow standard precautions. Wear gloves or use a protective barrier to prevent contamination from the blood.

   b. Position the victim flat on the back. Separate the legs to prevent pressure on the genital area.

   c. If any tissue is torn from the area, preserve the tissue by placing it in cool, sterile water or normal saline solution or in gauze moistened with sterile water. Put the tissue on ice and send it to the medical facility along with the victim.

   d. Apply cold compresses such as covered ice bags to the area to relieve pain and reduce swelling.

   e. Obtain medical help for the victim.

10. Be alert for signs of shock in all victims. Treat for shock immediately.

11. Constantly reassure all victims while providing care. Remain calm. Encourage the victim to relax as much as possible.

12. Always obtain medical help as quickly as possible. Shock, pain, and injuries to vital organs can cause death in a very short period of time.

Practice *Use the evaluation sheet for 13:10, Providing First Aid for Specific Injuries, to practice this procedure. When you feel you have mastered this skill, sign the sheet and give it to your instructor for further action.*

✔ **Final Checkpoint** Using the criteria listed on the evaluation sheet, your instructor will grade your performance.

Name _____ Date _____

Evaluated by _____

DIRECTIONS: Practice providing first aid for specific injuries according to the criteria listed. When you are ready for your final check, give this sheet to your instructor.

Providing First Aid for Specific Injuries	Points Possible	Yes	No	Points Earned	Comments
1. Follows priorities of care:					
Checks the scene	1				
Checks consciousness and breathing	1				
Calls emergency medical services	1				
Cares for victim	1				
Controls bleeding	1				
2. Observes victim for signs and symptoms of specific injuries	2				
3. Provides first aid for *eye injuries* as follows:					
Washes hands thoroughly	2				
Removes free-floating foreign object:					
Draws upper lid down over lower lid	2				
Raises upper lid and removes object with sterile gauze or gently flushes eye with water	2				
Applies sterile dressing if object is embedded or above techniques do not work on free-floating object	2				
If an object is protruding from the eye, immobilizes with dressings or cup with hole in bottom and makes no attempt to remove	2				
Covers both eyes with dressings to prevent movement of injured eye	2				
Positions victim lying flat	2				
Obtains medical help	2				
4. Provides first aid for *ear injuries* as follows:					
Applies light pressure with sterile dressing to control bleeding	2				
Preserves torn tissue by putting it in sterile water or normal saline or gauze moistened with sterile water or normal saline	2				
Places sterile gauze loosely in outer ear canal for perforation of eardrum	2				
If cerebrospinal fluid is draining from ear:					
Avoids any attempt to stop flow	2				
Positions victim on injured side with head and shoulders elevated slightly	2				
Positions dressing to absorb flow	2				
Obtains medical help	2				

Providing First Aid for Specific Injuries	Points Possible	Yes	No	Points Earned	Comments
5. Provides first aid for *brain injuries* as follows:					
Positions victim lying flat	2				
Elevates head and shoulders if no neck/spine injury	2				
Watches closely for respiratory distress	2				
Allows cerebrospinal fluid to drain and absorbs with dressings	2				
Avoids fluids—moistens lips, tongue, and mouth with cool, wet cloth if necessary	2				
Notes length of time the victim is unconscious	2				
Obtains medical help	2				
6. Provides first aid for *nosebleed* as follows:					
Positions victim sitting with head leaning slightly forward	2				
Presses bleeding nostril(s) to midline	2				
If bleeding does not stop, inserts gauze in nostril(s) and applies pressure	2				
Applies cold, wet compress or covered ice bag to bridge of nose	2				
Obtains medical help if bleeding does not stop, fracture suspected, or victim has repeated nosebleeds	2				
7. Provides first aid for *chest injuries* as follows:					
For sucking chest wound:					
Applies airtight dressing using aluminum foil or plastic wrap and tapes on 3 sides	3				
Positions victim on injured side and elevates head and chest slightly	2				
For penetrating object:					
If object protruding, immobilizes in place and makes no attempt to remove it	3				
Positions victim in comfortable position but avoids unnecessary movement	2				
Watches closely for respiratory distress	2				
Obtains medical help immediately	2				
8. Provides first aid for *abdominal injuries* as follows:					
Positions victim lying flat with knees flexed slightly	2				
Elevates head and shoulders slightly to aid breathing	2				
If organs protruding, covers organs with sterile dressing moistened with sterile water or normal saline and plastic wrap or foil	3				
Avoids giving oral fluids	2				
Obtains medical help immediately	2				

Evaluation 13:10 (cont.)

Providing First Aid for Specific Injuries	Points Possible	Yes	No	Points Earned	Comments
9. Provides first aid for *injuries to genital organs* as follows:					
Controls bleeding with direct pressure	2				
Positions victim lying flat with legs separated	2				
Preserves any torn tissue by placing it in cool, sterile water or normal saline or in gauze moistened with cool, sterile water or normal saline	2				
Applies cold compresses or covered ice bag	2				
Obtains medical help	2				
10. Observes all victims for signs of shock and treats for shock immediately	2				
11. Reassures victim while providing care; encourages victim to relax as much as possible	2				
Totals	100				

13:11 PROVIDING FIRST AID FOR SUDDEN ILLNESS

ASSIGNMENT SHEET

Grade _____ Name _____

INTRODUCTION: Sudden illness can occur in any individual, and you should know the major facts regarding first aid. This assignment will help you review these facts.

INSTRUCTIONS: Review the information on Providing First Aid for Sudden Illness. In the space provided, print the word(s) that best completes the statement or answers the question.

1. Identify two (2) sources of information you can use to help determine what illness a victim has.

2. List three (3) signs and symptoms of a heart attack.

3. List two (2) first aid treatments for a heart attack victim.

4. List four (4) signs and symptoms of a stroke.

5. List two (2) first aid treatments for a stroke.

6. If early symptoms of fainting are noted, how should you position the victim?

7. List two (2) points of first aid care for a victim who has fainted.

8. What is a convulsion?

9. First aid care for the victim with a convulsion is directed at preventing _____.

10. Should a padded tongue blade or soft object be placed between the victim's teeth during a convulsion? Why or why not?

11. Why is it important not to use force or restrain the muscle movements during a convulsion?

12. In a victim with diabetes, an increase in the level of glucose or sugar in the blood can lead to a condition called _____, and an excess amount of insulin can lead to a condition called _____.

13. List four (4) signs and symptoms of diabetic coma.

14. What is the main treatment for diabetic coma?

15. List four (4) signs and symptoms of insulin shock.

16. What is the main treatment for insulin shock?

Equipment and Supplies

Blankets, pillows, sugar, clean cloth, cool water, disposable gloves

Procedure

1. Follow the priorities of care, if indicated.

   a. Check the scene. Move the victim only if absolutely necessary.

   b. Check the victim for consciousness and breathing.

   c. Call emergency medical services (EMS), if necessary.

   d. Provide care to the victim.

   e. Check for bleeding. Control severe bleeding.

   CAUTION: Follow standard precautions. If possible, wear gloves or use a protective barrier while controlling bleeding.

2. Closely observe the victim for specific signs and symptoms. If the victim is conscious, obtain information about the history of the illness, type and amount of pain, and other pertinent details. If the victim is unconscious, check for a medical bracelet or necklace or a medical information card. Always have a reason for everything you do. Explain your actions to any observers, especially if it is necessary to check the victim's wallet for a medical card.

3. If you suspect the victim is having a *heart attack*, provide first aid as follows:

   a. Place the victim in the most comfortable position possible but avoid unnecessary movement. Some victims will want to lie flat, but others will want to be in a partial or complete sitting position. If the victim is having difficulty breathing, use pillows or rolled blankets to elevate the head and shoulders.

   b. Obtain medical help for the victim immediately. Advise EMS that oxygen may be necessary.

   c. Encourage the victim to relax. Reassure the victim. Remain calm and encourage others to remain calm.

   d. Watch for signs of shock and treat for shock as necessary. Avoid overheating the victim.

   e. If the victim complains of excessive thirst, use a wet cloth to moisten the lips, tongue, and inside of the mouth. Small sips of water can also be given to the victim, but avoid giving large amounts of fluid.

   CAUTION: Do *not* give the victim ice water or very cold water because the cold can intensify shock.

4. If you suspect that the victim has had a *stroke*:

   a. Place the victim in a comfortable position. Keep the victim lying flat or slightly elevate the victim's head and shoulders to aid breathing. If the victim has difficulty swallowing, turn the victim on his or her side to allow secretions to drain from the mouth and prevent choking on the secretions.

   b. Reassure the victim. Encourage the victim to relax.

   c. Avoid giving the victim any fluids or food by mouth. If the victim complains of excessive thirst, use a cool, wet cloth to moisten the lips, tongue, and inside of the mouth.

   d. Obtain medical help for the victim as quickly as possible.

5. If the victim has *fainted*:

   a. Keep the victim in a supine position (that is, lying flat on the back). Raise the legs and feet 12 inches.

   b. Check for breathing. Provide artificial respiration, if necessary.

   c. Loosen any tight clothing.

   d. Use cool water to gently bathe the face.

Procedure 13:11 (cont.)

    e. Check for any other injuries.

    f. Encourage the victim to continue lying down until his or her skin color improves.

    g. If no other injuries are suspected, allow the victim to get up slowly. First, elevate the head and shoulders. Then place the victim in a sitting position. Allow the victim to stand slowly. If any signs of dizziness, weakness, or pallor are noted, return the victim to the supine position.

    h. If the victim does not recover quickly, or if any other injuries occur, obtain medical care. If fainting has occurred frequently, refer the victim for medical care.
       NOTE: Fainting can be a sign of a serious illness or condition.

6. If the victim is having a *convulsion*:

    a. Remove any dangerous objects from the area. If the victim is near heavy furniture or machinery that cannot be moved, move the victim to a safe area.

    b. Place soft material such as a blanket, small pillow, rolled jacket, or other similar material under the victim's head to prevent injury.

    c. Closely observe respirations at all times. During the convulsion, there will be short periods of apnea (cessation of breathing).
       NOTE: If breathing does not resume quickly, artificial respiration may be necessary.

    d. Do *not* try to place anything between the victim's teeth. This can cause injury to the teeth and/or gums.

    e. Do *not* attempt to restrain the muscle contractions.

    f. Note how long the convulsion lasts and what parts of the body are involved. Be sure to report this information to the EMS personnel.

    g. After the convulsion ends, closely watch the victim. Encourage the victim to rest.

    h. Obtain medical assistance if the seizure lasts more than a few minutes, if the victim has repeated seizures, if other severe injuries are apparent, if the victim does not have a history of seizures, or if the victim does not regain consciousness.

7. If the victim is in *diabetic coma*:

    a. Place the victim in a comfortable position. If the victim is unconscious, position him or her on either side to allow secretions to drain from the mouth.

    b. Frequently check respirations. Provide artificial respiration as needed.

    c. Obtain medical help immediately so the victim can be transported to a medical facility.

8. If the victim is in *insulin shock*:

    a. If the victim is conscious and can swallow, offer a drink containing sugar.

    b. If the victim is unconscious, place a small amount of granulated sugar under the victim's tongue.

    c. Place the victim in a comfortable position. Position an unconscious victim on either side to allow secretions to drain from the mouth.

    d. If recovery is not prompt, obtain medical help immediately.

9. Observe all victims of sudden illness for signs of shock. Treat for shock as necessary.

10. Constantly reassure any victim of sudden illness. Encourage relaxation to decrease stress.

Practice *Use the evaluation sheet for 13:11, Providing First Aid for Sudden Illness, to practice this procedure. When you feel you have mastered this skill, sign the sheet and give it to your instructor for further action.*

✔ **Final Checkpoint** Using the criteria listed on the evaluation sheet, your instructor will grade your performance.

Name _____ Date _____

Evaluated by _____

DIRECTIONS: Practice providing first aid for sudden illness according to the criteria listed. When you are ready for your final check, give this sheet to your instructor.

Providing First Aid for Sudden Illness	Points Possible	Yes	No	Points Earned	Comments
1. Follows priorities of care:					
Checks the scene	2				
Checks consciousness and breathing	2				
Calls emergency medical services	2				
Cares for victim	2				
Controls bleeding	2				
2. Observes victim for specific signs and symptoms of sudden illness	3				
3. Obtains information from victim regarding illness	3				
4. Checks for medical bracelet, necklace, or card if victim is unconscious	3				
5. Provides first aid for *heart attack* as follows:					
Positions victim in most comfortable position for victim	3				
Encourages relaxation	2				
Watches for signs of shock and treats as needed	2				
Moistens lips and mouth with wet cloth or gives small sips of water but avoids ice or cold water	2				
Obtains medical help as quickly as possible	2				
6. Provides first aid for *stroke* as follows:					
Positions in comfortable position	2				
Elevates head and shoulders to aid breathing	2				
Positions on side if victim is having difficulty swallowing or is unconscious	2				
Reassures victim and encourages relaxation	2				
Avoids fluids—moistens lips and mouth if necessary	2				
Obtains medical help immediately	2				

Evaluation 13:11 (cont.)

Providing First Aid for Sudden Illness	Points Possible	Yes	No	Points Earned	Comments
7. Provides first aid for *fainting* as follows:					
Keeps victim lying flat with feet raised if possible	3				
Loosens tight clothing on victim	2				
Bathes victim's face with cool water	2				
Checks for other injuries	2				
Encourages victim to lie flat until color improves	2				
After recovery, allows victim to get up slowly	3				
Obtains medical help if recovery is delayed, other injuries are noted, or other instances of fainting occur	2				
8. Provides first aid for *convulsions* as follows:					
Removes dangerous objects or moves victim if objects are too heavy to move	3				
Places pillow, blanket, or soft object under victim's head	3				
Checks respirations	2				
Avoids restraining muscle movements	2				
Notes length of convulsion and parts of body involved	2				
Watches closely after convulsion ends	2				
Obtains medical assistance if necessary	2				
9. Provides first aid for *diabetic coma* as follows:					
Positions victim in comfortable position or on side if unconscious	3				
Checks respirations	3				
Obtains medical help immediately	3				
10. Provides first aid for *insulin shock* as follows:					
Gives conscious victim drink with sugar	3				
Places sugar under tongue of unconscious victim	3				
Positions victim in comfortable position or on side if unconscious	3				
Obtains medical help if recovery not prompt	2				
11. Observes for signs of shock and treats as needed	3				
12. Reassures victim while providing care	3				
Totals	100				

13:12 APPLYING DRESSINGS AND BANDAGES

ASSIGNMENT SHEET

Grade _____ Name _____

INTRODUCTION: This assignment will help you review the main facts on dressings and bandages.

INSTRUCTIONS: Review the information on Applying Dressings and Bandages. In the space provided, print the word(s) that best completes the statement or answers the question.

1. What is a dressing?

2. List two (2) purposes or functions of dressings.

3. Why should you avoid using fluff cotton as a dressing?

4. What are bandages?

5. Bandages should be applied snugly enough to control _____ and prevent _____, but not so tightly that they interfere with _____.

6. List three (3) types or examples of bandages.

7. List three (3) uses for triangular bandages.

8. Why are elastic bandages hazardous?

9. List four (4) signs that indicate poor circulation.

10. If any signs of impaired or poor circulation are noted after a bandage has been applied, what should you do?

PROCEDURE 13:12 APPLYING DRESSINGS AND BANDAGES

Equipment and Supplies

Sterile gauze pads, triangular bandage, roller gauze bandage, elastic bandage, tape, disposable gloves

Procedure

1. Assemble equipment.

2. Wash hands. Put on gloves if there is any chance of contact with blood or body fluids.

3. *Apply a dressing to a wound* as follows:
   a. Obtain the correct size dressing. The dressing should be large enough to extend at least 1 inch beyond the edges of the wound.
   b. Open the sterile dressing package, taking care not to touch or handle the sterile dressing with your fingers.
   c. Use a pinching action to pick up the sterile dressing so you handle only one part of the outside of the dressing.
   d. Place the dressing on the wound. The untouched (sterile) side of the dressing should be placed on the wound. Do *not* slide the dressing into position. Instead, hold the dressing directly over the wound and then lower the dressing onto the wound.
   e. Secure the dressing in place with tape or with one of the bandage wraps.
      CAUTION: If tape is used, do not wrap it completely around the part. This can lead to impaired circulation.

4. *Apply a triangular bandage to the head or scalp:*
   a. Fold a 2-inch hem on the base (longest side) of the triangular bandage.
   b. Position and secure a sterile dressing in place over the wound.
   c. Keeping the hem on the outside, position the middle of the base of bandage on the forehead, just above the eyebrows.
   d. Bring the point of the bandage down over the back of the head.
   e. Bring the two ends of the base of the bandage around the head and above the ears. Cross the ends when they meet at the back of head. Bring them around to the forehead.
   f. Use a square knot to tie the ends in the center of the forehead.
   g. Use one hand to support the head. Use the other hand to gently but firmly pull down on the point of the bandage at the back of the head until the bandage is snug against the head.
   h. Bring the point up and tuck it into the bandage where the bandage crosses at the back of the head.

5. *Make a cravat bandage from a triangular bandage:*
   a. Bring the point of the triangular bandage down to the middle of the base (the long end of the bandage).
   b. Continue folding the bandage lengthwise until the desired width is obtained.

6. *Apply a circular bandage using a cravat bandage:*
   a. Place a sterile dressing on the wound.
   b. Place the center of the cravat bandage over the sterile dressing.
   c. Bring the ends of the cravat around the body part and cross them where they meet.
   d. Bring the ends back to the starting point.

Procedure 13:12 (cont.)

   e. Use a square knot to tie the ends of the cravat over the dressing.

       CAUTION: Avoid tying or wrapping the bandage too tightly. This could impair circulation.

       NOTE: Roller gauze bandage can also be used.

       CAUTION: This type of wrap is *never* used around the neck because it could strangle the victim.

7. *Apply a spiral wrap* using roller gauze bandage or elastic bandage:

   a. Place a sterile dressing over the wound.

   b. Hold the roller gauze or elastic bandage so that the loose end is hanging off the bottom of the roll.

   c. Start at the farthest end (the bottom of the limb) and move in an upward direction.

   d. Anchor the bandage by placing it on an angle at the starting point. To do this, encircle the limb once, leaving a corner of the bandage uncovered. Turn down this free corner and then encircle the part again with the bandage.

   e. Continue encircling the limb. Use a spiral type of motion to move up the limb. Overlap each new turn approximately one-half the width of the bandage.

   f. Use one or two circular turns to finish the wrap at the end point.

   g. Secure the end by taping, pinning, or tying. To avoid injury when pins are used, place your hand under the double layer of bandage and between the pin and the skin before inserting the pin. The end of the bandage can also be cut in half. The two halves are then brought around opposite sides and tied into place.

8. Use roller gauze bandage or elastic bandage to *apply a figure-eight ankle wrap*:

   a. Position a dressing over the wound.

   b. Anchor the bandage at the instep of the foot.

   c. Make one or two circular turns around the instep and foot.

   d. Bring the bandage up over the foot in a diagonal direction. Bring it around the back of the ankle and then down over the top of the foot. Circle it under the instep. This creates the figure-eight pattern.

   e. Repeat the figure-eight pattern. With each successive turn, move downward and backward toward the heel. Overlap the previous turn by one-half to two-thirds the width of the bandage.

       NOTE: Hold the bandage firmly but do not pull it too tightly. If you are using elastic bandage, avoid stretching the material during the application.

   f. Near completion, use one or two final circular wraps to circle the ankle.

   g. Secure the bandage in place by taping, pinning, or tying the ends.

       CAUTION: To avoid injury to the victim when pins are used, place your hand between the bandage and the victim's skin.

9. Use roller gauze bandage to *apply a recurrent wrap* to the fingers:

   a. Place a sterile dressing over the wound.

   b. Hold the roller gauze bandage so that the loose end is hanging off the bottom of the roll.

   c. Place the end of the bandage on the bottom of the finger. Then bring the bandage up to the tip of the finger and down to the bottom of the opposite side of the finger. With overlapping wraps, fold the bandage backward and forward over the finger three or four times.

   d. Start at the bottom of the finger and use a spiral wrap up and down the finger to hold the recurrent wraps in position.

   e. Complete the bandage by using a figure-eight wrap around the wrist. Bring the bandage in a diagonal direction across the back of the hand. Circle the wrist at least two times. Bring the bandage back over the top of the hand and circle the bandaged finger. Repeat this figure-eight motion at least twice.

   f. Secure the bandage by circling the wrist once or twice. Tie the bandage at the wrist.

Procedure 13:12 (cont.)

10. After any bandage has been applied, check the circulation below the bandage at frequent intervals. Note any signs of impaired circulation, including swelling, coldness, numbness or tingling, pallor or cyanosis, and poor return of pink color after nail beds are blanched by lightly pressing on them. If any signs of poor circulation are noted, loosen the bandages immediately.

11. Obtain medical help for any victim who may need additional care.

12. Remove gloves and wash hands.

Practice *Use the evaluation sheet for 13:12, Applying Dressings and Bandages, to practice this procedure. When you feel you have mastered this skill, sign the sheet and give it to your instructor for further action.*

✔ **Final Checkpoint** Using the criteria listed on the evaluation sheet, your instructor will grade your performance.

Name _____ Date _____

Evaluated by _____

DIRECTIONS: Practice applying dressings and bandages according to the criteria listed. When you are ready for your final check, give this sheet to your instructor.

Applying Dressings and Bandages	Points Possible	Yes	No	Points Earned	Comments
1. Assembles supplies	1				
2. Washes hands and puts on gloves	1				
3. Applies dressing as follows:					
Obtains correct size dressing	2				
Opens package without touching dressing	2				
Uses pinching action to pick up dressing	2				
Touches only one part of outside	2				
Holds dressing over wound and lowers onto wound	2				
Secures dressing with tape of bandage	2				
4. Applies triangular bandage to head or scalp as follows:					
Folds 2-inch hem in base	2				
Places sterile dressing on wound	2				
Positions middle of base on forehead with hem on outside	2				
Brings ends around head, above ears, crosses in back, and returns to forehead	2				
Ties ends in center of forehead with square knot	2				
Supports head while pulling point down in back to make bandage snug	2				
Tucks point into area where bandage crosses in back	2				
5. Folds a cravat with a triangular bandage as follows:					
Brings point down to base	2				
Folds lengthwise until desired width obtained	2				
6. Applies circular bandage using a cravat as follows:					
Places sterile dressing on wound	2				
Places center of cravat over dressing	2				
Carries ends around area and crosses where they meet	2				
Brings ends back to starting point	2				
Ties ends with square knot	2				

Applying Dressings and Bandages	Points Possible	Yes	No	Points Earned	Comments
7. Applies spiral wrap with roller gauze as follows:					
Places sterile dressing on wound	2				
Holds bandage with loose end coming off bottom	2				
Starts at bottom of limb and moves upward	2				
Anchors bandage correctly	2				
Circles area with spiral motion	2				
Overlaps each turn ½ width of bandage	2				
Ends with 1 or 2 circular turns around limb	2				
Secures with tape, pins, or by tying	2				
8. Applies figure-eight wrap as follows:					
Places sterile dressing on wound	2				
Anchors bandage on instep	2				
Circles foot once or twice	2				
Angles over top of foot	2				
Goes behind ankle	2				
Circles down over top of foot and under instep	2				
Repeats pattern, overlapping each turn ½ to ⅔ width of bandage	2				
Ends with 1 or 2 circular wraps around ankle	2				
Secures with tape, pins, or by tying	2				
9. Applies bandage to finger as follows:					
Places dressing on wound	2				
Holds gauze with loose end coming off bottom of roll	2				
Overlaps bandage on finger with 3 or 4 recurrent folds	2				
Uses spiral wrap to hold folds in position	2				
Uses figure-eight wrap around wrist to secure	2				
Ends by circling wrist	2				
Ties at wrist	2				
10. Checks circulation in area below bandage by noting following points:					
Pale or bluish	1				
Swelling	1				
Coldness	1				
Numbness or tingling	1				
Poor return of color after nail beds pressed lightly	1				
11. Loosens bandage immediately if any signs of impaired circulation noted	2				
12. Obtains medical help for victim as soon as possible	2				
13. Removes gloves and washes hands	1				
Totals	100				

CHAPTER 13 INTERNET SEARCHES

Use the suggested search engines in Chapter 9:4 of the textbook to search the Internet for additional information on the following topics:

1. *Organizations:* Find web sites for the American Red Cross, the American Heart Association, Emergency Medical Services, and Poison Control Centers to learn what services are offered.

2. *CPR:* Look for sites that discuss the principles of cardiopulmonary resuscitation, abdominal thrusts or the Heimlich maneuver, and cardiac emergencies.

3. *Automated External Defibrillators:* Search for manufacturers of AEDs and compare models.

4. *First aid treatments:* Find information on recommended treatment for bleeding, wounds, shock, poisoning, snakebites, insect stings, tick bites, burns, heat exposure, heat stroke, hypothermia, frostbite, fractures, dislocations, sprains, strains, eye injuries, nose injuries, head and skull injuries, spine injuries, chest injuries, abdominal injuries, myocardial infarction, cerebrovascular accident, fainting, convulsions or seizures, diabetic coma, and insulin shock.

CHAPTER 14 PREPARING FOR THE WORLD OF WORK

14:1 DEVELOPING JOB-KEEPING SKILLS

ASSIGNMENT SHEET

Grade _____ Name _____

INTRODUCTION: To keep a job, it will be essential for you to learn job-keeping skills. This assignment will help you evaluate your job-keeping skills.

INSTRUCTIONS: Read the information on Developing Job-Keeping Skills. In the space provided, print the word(s) that best completes the statement or answers the question.

1. Identify five (5) deficiencies that employers feel are common in high school students.

2. Choose at least two (2) job-keeping skills you feel you have. Give at least two (2) reasons why you feel you are competent in each of the skills.

3. Choose at least two (2) job-keeping skills for which you feel you need improvement. Explain why you are not competent in these skills. Then identify at least two (2) ways you can improve your competency in each of these skills.

14:2 WRITING A LETTER OF APPLICATION AND PREPARING A RESUMÉ

ASSIGNMENT SHEET

Grade _____ Name _____

INTRODUCTION: A letter of application and a resumé are two important parts of obtaining employment. This assignment will help you review the main facts regarding the letter and resumé.

INSTRUCTIONS: Read the information on Writing a Letter of Application and Preparing a Resumé. In the space provided, print the word(s) that best completes the statement or answers the question.

1. What is the main purpose of the letter of application?

2. Briefly state the contents for each of the paragraphs in a letter of application.

   a. paragraph 1:

   b. paragraph 2:

   c. paragraph 3:

   d. paragraph 4:

3. What is a resumé?

4. Briefly list the type of information found in each of the following parts of a resumé.

   a. personal identification:

   b. employment objective:

   c. educational background:

   d. work or employment experience:

   e. skills:

   f. other activities:

   g. references:

5. Why is honesty always the best policy when completing resumés?

6. What type of envelope should you use to mail the letter of application and resumé?

7. What is the purpose of a career passport or portfolio?

   List three (3) items that might be included in a career passport or portfolio.

8. List the three (3) foundation skills recognized by SCANS.

9. Choose two (2) of the SCANS workplace competencies. For each competency, write a brief explanation of how you have mastered it.

ASSIGNMENT SHEET

Grade _____ Name _____

INTRODUCTION: The following information is required for resumés.

INSTRUCTIONS: Use a telephone book, address books, school records, and other sources to complete the following information about yourself.

Name _____

Address _____
           Number & Street   City   State   Zip

Telephone (___) _____ Social Security _____

Name of School _____

School Address _____
               Number & Street   City   State   Zip

Dates of Attendance _____

Degree Earned _____ Major _____

Special Skills Learned _____

Computer Skills/Courses _____

Grade Average _____ Awards Earned _____

_____

_____

Other Schools Attended: Name _____

       Address _____

Previous Employers: Most recent first

Names	Address City, State, Zip	Dates of Employment	Duties Job Titles

References: Names (at least 3)   Full Address and Telephone   Title

_____

_____

_____

Other Activities: Include clubs, offices, volunteer work, hobbies

_____

_____

_____

Equipment and Supplies

Good-quality paper, inventory sheet for resumés, computer with word processing software and a printer, or typewriter

Procedure

1. Assemble equipment.

2. Re-read the section on letters of application and resumés in the textbook.

3. Review the sample letters of application and resumés.

4. Complete the inventory sheet for resumés. Check dates for accuracy. Be sure that names are spelled correctly. Use the telephone book or other sources to check addresses and zip codes.

5. Carefully evaluate all your information. Determine the best method of presenting your information. Try different ways of writing your material. Do not hesitate to show several different versions to your instructor or others and get their opinions on which way seems best.

6. Type a rough draft of a letter of application. Follow the correct form for letters. Use correct spacing and margins. Check for correct spelling and punctuation.

7. Type a final letter of application. Be sure it contains the required information. Proofread the letter for spelling errors and other mistakes. If possible, ask someone else to proofread your letter and evaluate it.

8. Type a rough draft of your resumé. Arrange the information in an attractive manner. Be sure that spacing is standard throughout the resumé and margins are even on all sides.

9. Review your sample resumé. Reword any information, if necessary. Be sure all information is pertinent and concise. Ask your instructor or others for opinions regarding suggested changes.

10. Type your final resumé. Take care to avoid errors. If you are not a good typist, it might be wise to have someone else complete the final draft. Proofread the final copy, checking carefully for errors. If possible, ask someone else to proofread your resumé and evaluate it.

    NOTE: Resumés can be copies of the original, but be sure the copies are of good quality. Letters of application must be originals. They are individually tailored for each potential job and, therefore, are not copied.

11. Replace all equipment.

Practice *Use the evaluation sheets for 14:2, Writing a Letter of Application and Preparing a Resumé, to practice this procedure. When you feel you have mastered this skill, sign the sheets and give them to your instructor for further action. Also give your instructor your letter of application and resumé along with the evaluation sheets.*

✔**Final Checkpoint** Using the criteria listed on the evaluation sheets, your instructor will grade your letter of application and resumé.

Name _____ Date _____

Evaluated by _____

DIRECTIONS: Practice writing a letter of application according to the criteria listed. When you are ready for your final check, give this sheet to your instructor.

Writing a Letter of Application	Points Possible	Yes	No	Points Earned	Comments
1. Use good-quality paper	6				
2. Computer prints or types all information neatly and accurately	6				
3. Follows correct form for letters	6				
4. Completes contents of letter as follows:					
Addresses letter to correct individual	8				
States purpose for writing	8				
States position applying for	8				
Lists source of advertisement or referring person	8				
States why qualified	8				
States resumé enclosed or furnished on request	8				
Includes information on how employer can contact	8				
Asks for interview and thanks employer for considering application	8				
5. Spells all words correctly	6				
6. Punctuates all information and sentences correctly	6				
7. Uses complete sentences and correct grammar	6				
Totals	100				

Name _____ Date _____

Evaluated by _____

DIRECTIONS: Practice preparing a resumé according to the criteria listed. When you are ready for your final check, give this sheet to your instructor.

Preparing a Resumé	Points Possible	Yes	No	Points Earned	Comments
1. Uses good-quality paper	6				
2. Computer prints or types all information neatly and accurately	6				
3. Follows consistent format and spacing throughout resumé	6				
4. Includes all of the following information:					
Personal identification: name, address, telephone number	10				
Employment objective	10				
Educational background: name and address of school, special courses or training completed	10				
Work or employment experience: names and addresses of employers, dates employed, job titles, descriptions of duties in order from most recent backward	10				
Skills and specific knowledge	10				
Other activities: organizations, offices held, awards, volunteer work, hobbies, interests	10				
References: full name, title, and address or states "References will be furnished on request"	10				
5. Spells all words correctly	6				
6. Punctuates all information correctly	6				
Totals	100				

14:3 COMPLETING JOB APPLICATION FORMS

ASSIGNMENT SHEET 1

Grade _____ Name _____

INTRODUCTION: This assignment will help you review the main facts about completing job application forms.

INSTRUCTIONS: Read the information on Completing Job Application Forms. In the space provided, print the word(s) that best completes the statement or answers the question.

1. Why do employers use job application forms?

2. List two (2) reasons why you should read the application form completely before you fill in the information.

3. If questions do not apply to you, what should you put in the space provided for the answer to the question?

4. Why is it important to watch spelling and punctuation?

5. If the application does not state otherwise, it is best to type or _____. Use _____ if printing.

6. Why must all information be correct and truthful?

7. If a space is labeled "office use only," how do you complete this section? Why?

8. What should you do before using anyone's name as a reference?

9. What is the purpose of the wallet card?

10. Identify two (2) things you should look for when you proofread your completed application.

14:3 COMPLETING JOB APPLICATION FORMS: WALLET CARD

ASSIGNMENT SHEET 2

Grade _____ Name _____

INTRODUCTION: When you are looking for a job, you must be prepared. To be sure that you always have the needed information, it is wise to carry a "wallet card" with you. A sample form is given.

INSTRUCTIONS: Complete the information listed. This is information that can be used during job interviews, but most of the time it is required for application forms. The sheet can be glued to an index card and kept in your wallet for easy reference. The information may also be written on a small index card.

Social Security _____

Grade School Name _____

    Address _____ Zip _____

    Dates Attended _____

Junior High School Name _____

    Address _____ Zip _____

    Dates Attended _____

High School Name _____

    Address _____ Zip _____

    Dates Attended _____

Special Training—Major _____

Computer Skills/Courses _____

Activities _____

Special Skills _____

_____

Employment:

Dates	Name	Position	Full Address and Telephone	Salary

References: Include name, title, full address, telephone (Include at least 3)

_____

_____

_____

Other Facts _____

ASSIGNMENT SHEET 3

Grade _____ Name _____

INTRODUCTION: To obtain a job, you will probably have to complete an application form. The sample form that follows will help prepare you for this task.

INSTRUCTIONS: Review the information about Completing Job Application Forms. Complete the information on your "wallet card." Then use this information to complete the following form.

Health Careers Unlimited Application

Please type or print all information required. Be sure all information is accurate and complete.

Name in Full _____

Full Address _____

City _____ State _____ Zip _____

Social Security _____ Telephone _____

Position Desired _____

What prompted you to apply here? _____

When will you be available to start work? _____

Will you work (check if yes) any shift? _____ Holidays? _____

          Weekends? _____ Part-time? _____ Full-time? _____

Salary Expected _____ Registration Number _____

Education: (Circle last grade completed)

High School   1   2   3   4   Name _____

          From _____ Address in Full _____

          To _____ _____

College   1   2   3   4   Name _____

          From _____ Address in Full _____

          To _____ _____

Military Record: Branch of Service _____

          Date Entered _____ Date Discharged _____

          Discharge Status _____ Rank _____

Activities/Organizations/Special Skills _____

Computer Skills/Courses _____

Name _____

Employment Record (list most recent position first)

Name of Employer _____

Full Address _____

Telephone _____ Dates: From _____ To _____

Supervisor's Name _____

Average Salary _____ Job Title _____

Reason for Leaving _____

Name of Employer _____

Full Address _____

Telephone _____ Dates: From _____ To _____

Supervisor's Name _____

Average Salary _____ Job Title _____

Reason for Leaving _____

Name of Employer _____

Full Address _____

Telephone _____ Dates: From _____ To _____

Supervisor's Name _____

Average Salary _____ Job Title _____

Reason for Leaving _____

References: List names, titles, full address, and telephone

1. _____
   _____

2. _____
   _____

3. _____
   _____

I affirm that all of these statements are true and correct. I grant permission for verification of any of these facts.

Date _____ Signature _____

Do not write below this line:

Date Interviewed _____ Position _____

Salary _____ Starting Date _____ Initials _____

Equipment and Supplies

Typewriter, computer and scanner, or pen; wallet card (Assignment Sheet 2); sample application forms (Assignment Sheet 3)

Procedure

1. Assemble equipment. If a typewriter is used, be sure the ribbon is of good quality. If a scanner is available, scan the application form into a word-processing program on a computer. The application form can then be completed using the computer and printed on a printer.

2. Complete all information on the wallet card in Assignment 2. Check dates and be sure information is accurate. List full addresses, zip codes, and names.

3. Review the information on completing job application forms in the textbook. Read additional references, as needed.

4. Read the entire sample application form in Assignment 3. Be sure you understand the information requested for each part. Read all directions completely.

5. Unless otherwise directed, type all information requested. If a typewriter is not available, use a black ink pen to print all information.

6. Complete all areas of the form. Use "none" or "NA" as a reply to items that do not apply to you.

7. Take care not to write in spaces labeled "office use only" or "do not write below this line." Leave these areas blank.

8. In the space labeled "*signature*," sign your name. Note any statement that may be printed by the signature line. Be sure you are aware of what you are signing and the permission you may be giving. Most employers request permission to contact previous employers and/or references.

9. Recheck the entire application. Be sure information is correct and complete. Note and correct any spelling errors. Be sure you have answered all of the questions.

10. Replace all equipment.

Practice *Use the evaluation sheet for 14:3, Completing Job Application Forms, to practice this procedure. Obtain sample job application forms from your instructor or other sources. When you feel you have mastered this skill, sign the sheet and give it to your instructor for further action.*

✔ **Final Checkpoint** Using the criteria listed on the evaluation sheet, your instructor will grade your job application form.

Name _____ Date _____

Evaluated by _____

DIRECTIONS: Practice completing job application forms according to the criteria listed. When you are ready for your final check, give this sheet to your instructor.

Completing Job Application Forms	Points Possible	Yes	No	Points Earned	Comments
1. Completes wallet card correctly:					
Prints or types neatly	8				
Inserts accurate information	8				
Lists full addresses, zip codes, names, etc.	8				
2. Types or prints in black ink on application form unless writing requested on form	7				
3. Follows all directions provided on form	8				
4. Completes all of the following information on form:					
Personal information	8				
Education	8				
Work experience	8				
References	8				
Signature in correct area	8				
5. Spells all words correctly	7				
6. Leaves "office space" and similar areas blank	7				
7. Completes form neatly and thoroughly; places "none" or "NA" in spaces as necessary	7				
Totals	100				

14:4 PARTICIPATING IN A JOB INTERVIEW

ASSIGNMENT SHEET

Grade _____ Name _____

INTRODUCTION: A job interview is an essential part of obtaining a job. This assignment will review the main facts.

INSTRUCTIONS: Review the information on Participating in a Job Interview. In the space provided, print the word(s) that best completes the statement or answers the question.

1. List two (2) purposes of the job interview.

2. List two (2) things containing information that you should take to the job interview with you.

3. List three (3) rules for dress or appearance that should be observed.

4. How early should you arrive for a job interview?

5. List five (5) rules of conduct that should be observed during a job interview.

6. What should you do after the job interview to let the employer know you are still interested in the position?

7. Write a brief response to each of the following questions as though you were being asked during a job interview.

   a. "Why do you feel you are qualified for this position?"

   b. "What are your strengths or strong points?"

   c. "What do you hope to accomplish during the next two years?"

PROCEDURE 14:4 PARTICIPATING IN A JOB INTERVIEW

Equipment and Supplies

Desk, two chairs, evaluation sheets, lists of questions

Procedure

1. Assemble equipment. Role play a mock interview with four persons. Arrange for two people to evaluate the interview, one person to be the interviewer, and you to be the interviewee.

2. Position the two evaluators in such a way that they can observe both the interviewer and you, the person being interviewed. Make sure they will not interfere with the interview.

3. The interviewer should be seated at the desk and have a list of possible questions to ask during the interview.

4. Play the role of the person being interviewed. Prepare for this role by doing the following:
   - Be sure you have all necessary information. Prepare your wallet card, resumé, job application form, and/or career passport or portfolio.
   - Dress appropriately for the interview.
   - Arrive at least 5 to 10 minutes early for the interview.

5. When you are called for the interview, introduce yourself. Be sure to refer to the interviewer by name.

6. Sit in the chair indicated. Be aware of your posture. Be sure to sit straight. Keep your feet flat on the floor or cross your legs at the ankles only.

7. Listen carefully to the employer. Answer all questions thoroughly and completely. Think before you speak. Organize your information.

8. Maintain eye contact. Avoid distracting mannerisms.

9. Use correct grammar. Avoid slang expressions. Speak in complete sentences. Practice good manners.

10. When you are asked whether you have any questions, ask questions pertaining to the job responsibilities. Avoid a series of questions on salary, fringe benefits, vacations, time off, and so forth.

11. At the end of the interview, thank the interviewer for his or her time. Shake hands as you leave.

12. Check your performance by looking at the evaluation sheets completed by the two observers. Study suggested changes.

13. Replace all equipment.

Practice *Use the evaluation sheet for 14:4, Participating in a Job Interview, to practice this procedure. When you feel you have mastered this skill, sign the sheet and give it to your instructor for further action.*

✔**Final Checkpoint** Using the criteria listed on the evaluation sheet, your instructor will grade your performance.

Name _____ Date _____

Evaluated by _____

DIRECTIONS: Practice participating in a job interview according to the criteria listed. When you are ready for your final check, give this sheet to your instructor.

Participating in a Job Interview	Points Possible	Yes	No	Points Earned	Comments
1. Dresses appropriately for interview	6				
2. Prepares wallet card, resumé, job application	5				
3. Arrives 5–10 minutes early for interview	5				
4. Introduces self to employer and shakes hands firmly if indicated	5				
5. Refers to employer by name	5				
6. Sits correctly with good posture	5				
7. Listens carefully to the employer's questions and comments	6				
8. Answers all questions thoroughly but keeps answers pertinent	6				
9. Speaks slowly and clearly without mumbling	6				
10. Smiles when appropriate but avoid excessive laughter or giggling	5				
11. Maintains eye contact with employer	6				
12. Avoids distracting mannerisms during interview	6				
13. Uses correct English and avoids slang terms	6				
14. Uses correct manners and acts politely	6				
15. Avoids smoking, chewing gum, eating candy, and so forth	5				
16. Asks questions pertaining to job responsibility and avoids questioning fringe benefits, raises, and so forth	6				
17. Thanks employer for the interview at the end	6				
18. Shakes hands firmly if indicated	5				
Totals	100				

14:5 DETERMINING NET INCOME

ASSIGNMENT SHEET

Grade _____ Name _____

INTRODUCTION: To determine how much money you will have available after deductions, you must figure out your net income. This assignment will help you do this.

INSTRUCTIONS: Follow the instructions in each of the following sections. Place your answers in the blanks on the right. Double-check all figures for accuracy. Your instructor will supply an hourly wage rate if you are not employed.

1. List your wage per hour (how much you make in an hour).

    1. _____

2. Multiply your wage per hour times the number of hours you work per week. A 40-hour work week is an average amount.

    Wage Per Hour × Hours Worked Per Week =

    2. _____

    This amount is your gross weekly pay.

3. Determine the average deductions that will be taken out of your gross weekly pay.

   a. Determine the deduction for federal tax by multiplying gross pay times the percentage of deduction found on federal tax tables. (An average amount is 15% or 0.15.)

    _____ × _____ =
    Gross Pay   Federal Tax Percentage

    3. a. _____

   b. Determine the deduction for state tax by multiplying gross pay times the percentage of deduction found on state tax tables. (An average amount is 2% or 0.02.)

    _____ × _____ =
    Gross Pay   State Tax Percentage

    b. _____

   c. Determine the deduction for city/corporation tax by multiplying gross pay times the percentage found on city tax tables. (An average amount is 1% or 0.01.)

    _____ × _____ =
    Gross Pay   City Tax Percentage

    c. _____

   d. Determine the deduction for FICA or Social Security by multiplying gross pay times the current deduction. (Use 7.65% or 0.0765 if unknown.)

    _____ × _____ =
    Gross Pay   Social Security Percentage

    d. _____

e. List any other deductions that are subtracted from your gross pay. These deductions can include payments for insurance, charity, union dues, and so forth. Add all these deductions together to get the total for miscellaneous deductions.

e. _____

_____

_____

f. Add the answers in a., b., c., d., and e. together to get the total amount of deductions.

f. _____

4. Subtract the amount in answer 3.f. (total amount of all deductions) from the gross weekly pay listed in question 2. This amount will be your net weekly pay or "take home" weekly pay.

_____ − _____ = _____
Gross Pay   Deductions   Net Weekly Pay

4. _____

5. To determine your net pay per month, multiply the weekly net pay times 4 for four-week months. Multiply the weekly net pay times 5 for five-week months.

_____ × _____ = _____
Net Weekly Pay   Weeks per Month   Net Monthly Pay

5. _____

NOTE: The weekly net pay can be multiplied by 52 weeks to determine yearly net pay.

Equipment and Supplies

Assignment sheet for 14:5, Determining Net Income; pen or pencil

Procedure

1. Assemble equipment. If a calculator is available, you may use it to complete this assignment.

2. Read the instructions on the assignment sheet for 14:5, Determining Net Income.

3. Determine your wage per hour by using your salary in a current job or an amount assigned by your instructor. Multiply this amount by the number of hours you work per week. This is your gross weekly pay.

4. If your instructor provides tax tables, read the tax tables to determine the percentage, or amount of money, that will be withheld for federal tax. If tax tables are not available, check with your employer to obtain this information.

   NOTE: The average withholding tax for the lowest income bracket is approximately 15 percent. If you cannot find the exact amount or percentage, use this amount (0.15) for an approximate determination.

5. Multiply the percentage for federal tax times your gross weekly pay to determine the amount deducted for federal tax.

6. Determine the deduction for state tax by reading your state tax tables or by consulting your employer.

   NOTE: An average state tax is 2 percent. If you cannot find the exact amount or percentage, use this amount (0.02) for an approximate determination.

7. Multiply the percentage for state tax by your gross weekly pay to determine the amount deducted for state tax.

8. Determine the deduction for any city or corporation tax by reading the city/corporation tax tables or consulting your employer.

   NOTE: An average city/corporation tax is 1 percent. If you cannot find the exact amount or percentage, use this amount (0.01) for an approximate determination.

9. Multiply the percentage for city/corporation tax by your gross weekly pay to determine the amount deducted for city/corporation tax.

10. Check the current deduction for FICA, or Social Security and Medicare, by checking the tax tables or asking your employer for this information. Determine the deduction for FICA by multiplying your gross weekly pay by this percentage.

    NOTE: In 2002, the FICA rate was 6.2 percent of the first $84,900 in income and 1.45 percent of total income for Medicare. Use this total of 7.65 percent, or 0.0765, if you cannot obtain another percentage.

11. List the amounts for any other deductions. Examples include insurance, charitable donations, union dues, and similar items.

12. Add the amounts determined for federal tax, state tax, city/corporation tax, social security, and other deductions together.

13. Subtract the total amount for deductions from your gross weekly pay. The amount left is your net, or "take home," pay.

14. Recheck any figures, as needed.

15. Replace all equipment.

Practice *Use the evaluation sheet for 14:5, Determining Net Income. Practice determining net income according to the criteria listed on the evaluation sheet. When you feel you have mastered this skill, sign the sheet and give it to your instructor for further action.*

✔ **Final Checkpoint** Using the criteria listed on the evaluation sheet, your instructor will grade your performance.

Name _____ Date _____

Evaluated by _____

DIRECTIONS: Practice determining net income according to the criteria listed. When you are ready for your final check, give this sheet to your instructor.

Determining Net Income	Points Possible	Yes	No	Points Earned	Comments
1. Lists wage per hour	10				
2. Determines gross weekly pay by multiplying wage per hour times the number of hours worked per week	14				
3. Determines deduction for federal tax by multiplying correct percentage times gross weekly pay	10				
4. Determines deduction for state tax by multiplying correct percentage times gross weekly pay	10				
5. Determines deduction for city/corporation tax by multiplying correct percentage times gross weekly pay	10				
6. Determines deduction for social security by multiplying correct percentage times gross weekly pay	10				
7. Lists any miscellaneous deductions and obtains a total by adding all miscellaneous deductions together	10				
8. Adds amounts for federal tax, state tax, city/corporation tax, social security, and miscellaneous deductions together	12				
9. Subtracts total amount of deductions from gross weekly pay to get net weekly pay	14				
Totals	100				

14:6 CALCULATING A BUDGET

ASSIGNMENT SHEET

Grade _____ Name _____

INTRODUCTION: Avoiding financial problems requires planning. This assignment will help you prepare a budget and plan monthly expenses. Follow the instructions in each section to calculate a budget.

1. List monthly expenses for the following items:

   Rent (you may have to share an apartment) _____

   Utilities: heat, electricity, telephone, water, garbage removal, and so forth _____

   Food: include all food items purchased, money for food away from home _____

   Car expenses: _____

       Gasoline _____

       Insurance (divide yearly payment by 12) _____

       Oil, maintenance, tires, repairs _____

       Payment for purchase _____

       Other: (note what) _____

   Laundry or cleaning of clothes _____

   Clothing purchase (include uniforms) _____

   Payments: Furniture _____

               Charge accounts _____

               Other bills _____

   Personal items: shampoo, toothpaste, and so forth _____

   Donations: Church, charities _____

   Medical or life insurance payments (divide yearly payment by 12) _____

   Education expenses (fees, books, and so forth) _____

   Savings (strive for 10%) _____

   Other items: List _____ _____

                         _____ _____

   Entertainment, hobbies, and so forth _____

   Miscellaneous: "Mad" money, and so forth _____

                                          TOTAL 1. $ _____

2. List your net pay per four-week month.

                                          TOTAL 2. $ _____

3. If the total in number 2 is larger than the total in number 1, you may add more money to items in your budget. If number 1 is larger, you have overspent. Refigure your budget. The figure in number 1 should equal the figure in number 2 for a balanced budget.

Equipment and Supplies

Assignment sheet for 14:6, Calculating a Budget; pen or pencil

Procedure

1. Assemble equipment. If a calculator is available, you may use it to complete this procedure.

2. Read the instructions on the assignment sheet for 14:6, Calculating a Budget.

3. Determine your fixed expenses for a one-month period. This includes amounts you must pay for rent, utilities, loans, charge accounts, insurance, and similar items. List these expenses.

4. Determine your variable expenses for a one-month period. This includes amounts for clothing purchases, personal items, donations, entertainment, and similar items. List these expenses.

5. List any other items that must be included in your monthly budget. Be sure to list a reasonable amount for each item.

6. Determine a reasonable amount for savings. Many people prefer to set aside a certain percentage of their net monthly pay as savings.

7. Determine your net monthly pay. Double check all figures for accuracy.

8. Add all of your monthly budget expenses together. This sum represents your total expenditures per month.

9. Compare your expense total to your net monthly income. If your expense total is higher than your net income, you will have to revise your budget and reduce any expenses that are not fixed. If your expense total is lower than your net income, you may increase the dollar amounts of your budget items. If the other figures in your budget are realistic, it may be wise to increase the dollar amount of savings.

10. When the expense total in your budget equals your monthly net income, you have a balanced budget. Live by this budget and avoid any expenditures not listed on the budget.

11. Replace all equipment.

Practice *Use the evaluation sheet for 14:6, Calculating a Budget, to practice this procedure. When you feel you have mastered this skill, sign the sheet and give it to your instructor for further action. Give your instructor a completed budget along with the evaluation sheet.*

✔ **Final Checkpoint** Using the criteria listed on the evaluation sheet, your instructor will grade your budget.

Name _____ Date _____

Evaluated by _____

DIRECTIONS: Practice calculating a budget according to the criteria listed. When you are ready for your final check, give this sheet to your instructor.

Calculating a Budget	Points Possible	Yes	No	Points Earned	Comments
1. Lists realistic monthly amounts for each of the following items:					
Rent or house payments	5				
Utilities	5				
Food	5				
Car expenses:					
Gasoline	3				
Insurance (divides yearly payment by 12)	3				
Oil, maintenance, and so forth	3				
Payment for purchase	3				
Laundry or cleaning of clothes	5				
Clothing purchase	5				
Payments:					
Furniture	3				
Charge accounts	3				
Other bills	3				
Personal items	5				
Donations	5				
Medical or life insurance (divides yearly payments by 12)	5				
Education expenses	5				
Savings	5				
Entertainment, hobbies	5				
Miscellaneous expenses	5				
2. Determines accurate net monthly income	6				
3. Calculates an accurate total for monthly expenses	6				
4. Balances budget by making monthly expenses equal net monthly income	7				
Totals	100				

CHAPTER 14 INTERNET SEARCHES

Use the suggested search engines in Chapter 9:4 of the textbook to search the Internet for additional information on the following topics:

1. *Components of a job search:* Find information on letters of application or cover letters, resumés, job interviews, and job application forms.

2. *Requirements of employers:* Locate information on skills and qualities that employers desire.

3. *Job search:* Look for sites that provide information on employment opportunities. For specific health care careers, look for opportunities under organizations for the specific career. Also check general sites such as *monster.com*, *job-listing.com*, *jobsleuth.com*, and *joblocator.com*.

4. *Salary and wages:* Check sites such as the Internal Revenue Service (IRS), state and local tax departments, and Social Security Administration for information on taxes and tax rates. Also locate sites on money management, budgeting, and financial management for information on how to manage money.

INDEX

Abbreviations, 115–117
Abdominal injuries, 251, 254, 256
Accidents, preventing, 132–136
Admission form, 48–55
Ambulation, crutches, 83–90
Aneroid sphygmomanometer, 190
Apical pulse, 184–186
Application
  forms, 278–283
  letter, 272–273, 275, 276
Aseptic techniques, 145–162
Assessment, personal, 65–68
Aural temperature, 175–177

Bandages, 264–269
Bioterrorism, 163
Bleeding, 214–219
Blood and body fluid precautions, 151–156
Blood pressure, 187–193
Body mechanics, 129–131
Bone injuries, 243–249
Brain injuries, 250–251, 253, 256
Brushing teeth, 19–23
Budget, 291–293
Burns, 230–234

Cardiopulmonary resuscitation, 197–213
Careers, health care, 15–18
Chest injuries, 251, 253, 256
Child CPR, 205–207
Choking, 208–213
Clinical thermometer, 170–172
Cold exposure, 240–242
Coma, diabetic, 259, 261, 263
Communications, 9–13
Compress, moist, 91–96
Computers, 127–128
Convulsions, 259, 261, 263
CPR, 197–213
Cravat bandage, 265, 268
Crutches, 83–90
Cultural diversity, 109–113

Data sheet, statistical, 41–47
Diabetes, 259, 261, 263
Dressings, 264–269

Ear injuries, 250–251, 252–253, 255–256
Effective communications, 9–13
Electronic thermometer, 173–174
Ethical responsibilities, 103–107
Evaluation sheet, description, vii–viii

Examination, safety, 141–143
Eye injuries, 250, 252, 255

Facilities, health care, 5–7
Fainting, 258–259, 260–261, 263
Feeding patient, 77–82
Figure–eight wrap, 266, 269
Fire safety, 137–140
First aid, 195–270
Flossing teeth, 19–20, 24–25
Frostbite, 240–242

Genital injuries, 254, 257
Gross income, 287–290

Hand washing, 148–150
Health care
  careers, 15–18
  history, 1–4
  facilities, 5–7
  skill standards, x–xiv
  systems, 5–7
  trends, 1–4
  worker, 9–13
Heart attack, 258, 260, 262
Heat exposure, 235–239
Height, measuring, 56–61
History, health care, 1–4

Illness, 258–263
Income, 287–290
Infant CPR, 202–204
Infection control, 145–162
Injuries
  first aid, 214–219, 243–249, 250–257
  preventing, 132–136
Insect bite, 227, 229
Insulin shock, 259, 261, 263
Internet searches, 4, 7, 13, 102, 107, 114, 122, 125, 128, 144, 164, 194, 270, 294
Interview, job, 284–286
Inventory, resume, 274
Isolation, 157–162

Job
  applications, 278–283
  interview, 284–286
  keeping skills, 271
Joint injuries, 243–249

Legal responsibilities, 103–107
Letter of application, 272–273, 275, 276

Math, 123–125
Medical terminology, 118–121
Mental health myths, 62–64
Mercury sphygmomanometer, 189
Microscope, 26–33
Moist compress, 91–96

National Health Care Skill Standards, xiii–xiv
Net income, 287–290
Nosebleed, 251, 253, 256

Obituary, 69–70
Obstructed airway, 208–213
Oral temperature, 167–174
Organisms, classes of, 145–147
Oxygen, 34–40

Personal
    assessment, 65–68
    qualities, 9–13
Poisoning, 225–229
Prefixes, 118–121
Pulse
    apical, 184–186
    radial, 178–180

Radial pulse, 178–180
Recurrent wrap, 266, 269
Respiration, 181–183
Resume, 272–275, 277

Safety, 132–143
Screening vision, 97–101
Shock, 220–224
Skeletal injuries, 243–249
Sling, 244, 246, 248–249
Snakebite, 227, 229
Sphygmomanometer, 189–190

Spiral wrap, 266, 269
Splints, 244, 245–246, 248
Standard precautions, 151–156
Statistical data sheet, 41–47
Stroke, 258, 260, 262
Suffixes, 118–121
Systems health care, 5–7

Teeth, brushing and flossing, 19–23
Temperature, 167–177
Terminology, medical, 118–121
Test
    mental health, 62–64
    safety, 141–143
    vision, 97–101
Thermometer, 166–177
Transfer, wheelchair, 71–76
Transmission-based isolation, 157–162
Trends, health care, 1–4
Triangular bandage, 264, 265, 268
Tympanic temperature, 175–177

Universal precautions. See Standard precautions

Vision screening, 97–101
Vital signs, 165–194

Wallet card, 278, 279
Washing hands, 148–150
Weight, measuring, 56–61
Wheelchair transfer, 71–76
Word parts, 118–121
Wounds, 214–219
Writing
    letter of application, 272–273, 275, 276
    obituary, 69–70
    resume, 272–275, 277